A GIFT
OF COURAGE

A GIFT
OF COURAGE

Thomas S. Morse, M.D.

DOUBLEDAY & COMPANY, INC.

GARDEN CITY, NEW YORK

1982

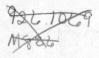

Library of Congress Cataloging in Publication Data

Morse, Thomas S.
    A gift of courage.

    Includes index.
    1. Morse, Thomas S.   2. Pediatric surgeons—
United States—Biography.   I. Title.
RD27.35.M66A34   617'.980924   [B]   AACR2
ISBN: 0-385-17777-1
Library of Congress Catalog Card Number 81-43733

For Patty—

my tender comrade through four years of medical school, seven years of medical and surgical training, and all the years beyond.

How empty and how different those years would have been without you, and how far short of the mark I would have fallen had you not been at my side!

Contents

A GIFT
OF COURAGE

1

Becoming a Doctor

One blustery December day I found a particularly terrified three-year-old boy quivering on my examining table. A veritable mountain of winter clothing was piled beside him. His mother had succeeded in divesting him of everything except his underpants. These he gripped with ten white knuckles, defying anyone in the world to take them down. But somehow, down they must come, because the purpose of his visit was to see if he had a hernia in his groin. His mother sat on a chair beside him looking up at me with a look of despair which seemed to say, "Doctor, I've done the very best I could, but he's *so* frightened."

Assuming complete control of the situation, I marched up to the little lad and said confidently, "Johnnie, I can tell you what you had for lunch." Johnnie didn't utter a sound, but the defiant look on his face clearly said, "No you can't." Rubbing his tummy gently in a neutral area well away from the disputed underpants, I announced after a grave pause, "Aha! P. and J."

The response to this pronouncement was most satisfactory. Clearly, this little boy had met a genius. There was no point in fighting a man who could tell just by rubbing your stomach that you had recently ingested peanut butter and jelly. Down came the underpants without further protest, and the necessary examination was quickly concluded.

"Well," I said triumphantly, "you had better get dressed now, hadn't you?" I've seen some pretty fast pants-puter-oners in my day, but this kid broke all records. He went from no underpants to full winter garb including snowsuit, galoshes, hat, scarf, and mittens in less than twenty seconds—all by himself. His mother sat there dumbfounded.

"Oh Doctor," she gushed, "you were so wonderful!"

I was about to say, "It's nothing, Mother, all kids his age eat peanut butter and jelly," when she added, "but you forgot to mention the apple he had for lunch!"

Looking him humbly in the eye, I admitted, "Johnnie, you sure did fool me, 'cause I didn't feel any apple at all in your tummy." Without lowering his gaze from mine, Johnnie slowly produced an apple from the depths of his snowsuit pocket and whispered solemnly, "I didn't eat it yet."

Surely rewards must come to physicians who care for adults, but what can compare to moments like these which enchant the life of a children's surgeon?

It was much easier to get into medical school in 1949 than it is today. Twenty years after I sailed easily into the Cornell Medical School I completed a six-year term on a medical school admissions committee. Every week from the beginning of September to the end of the following April we pored over college transcripts, Medical College Aptitude Test scores, and letters of recommendation. On the basis of these documents we eliminated half of each year's applicants. The remaining six hundred we interviewed. Each candidate was interviewed not once but three times, being required to match wits with a minimum of seven and often as many as ten medical college professors. Fully two thirds of those we interviewed were denied admission, not because we felt they wouldn't become good physicians, but because there were not enough places in the medical school to accommodate them. Every week we turned down candidates far better prepared for the rigors of medical school than any of us had been. I am absolutely convinced that no medical school would have admitted me had I applied twenty years later than I did.

The courses we took during the first two years were similar to the basic science courses we had taken in college and consisted of lectures, demonstrations, and laboratory exercises. We studied anatomy, chemistry, pathology, and bacteriology as if our lives depended on it. The same study skills we had used in college brought predictable results, and during the first two years the same students who had excelled in college were at the head of the medical school class. The sick patients in the hospital were only a few feet away, but during those first two years they might as well have been in another country. Our isolation from patients made it difficult for us to see ourselves as internists, surgeons, or family practitioners. It often seemed that we would never break out of the lecture-laboratory-demonstration routine into the world of living, breathing, suffering people.

The third and fourth years were as different from the first two as day is from night. No longer did all eighty-six of us assemble in a lecture hall in the morning and proceed together through a long day of didactics. We found ourselves divided into small groups of eight or ten, scattered throughout the great hospital. Some began on the medical wards, probably the most logical place to begin. Others began in the surgical clinics, still others on the pediatric wards, and so on. Sooner or later each group would touch all the bases, but at any point along the way our cumulative information was different from that of every other group. The surprising thing is that it doesn't seem to matter in what sequence medical students are exposed to the various medical and surgical disciplines. Those who watch surgeons perform operations before seeing how internists determine the need for surgery seem no better or worse for this apparently illogical order of march. Those who learn how to diagnose measles and chicken pox before ever seeing a baby born appear as competent as those who witness these phenomena in a more chronological sequence.

Most of us had not the faintest idea what sort of doctors we wanted to become. The few with fathers or other relatives in medicine had a huge advantage over the rest of us because they knew a little of what the life that lay ahead of us would be like. We envied them.

Our first encounters with actual patients were terrifying experiences. About all we knew how to do was to introduce ourselves optimistically as "Dr. Jones" and ask how the patient was feeling. Usually the patient indicated that he was feeling terrible and wanted to know what we were going to do about it. We hadn't the slightest idea what to do about it. Some of the patients had been around long enough to be wise to our ignorance, and a few took fiendish glee in confounding us. More than one greenhorn, upon asking what had brought a patient to the hospital, was blandly informed that he had come by taxi.

Gradually, painfully, and sometimes with pathetic humor, we learned how to talk to sick people, to ask the questions that ferret out the information needed to arrive at a diagnosis and to convey to them that we really were concerned about their problems and eager, if not always competent, to help them. As we lost our dread of these encounters we began to enjoy the feeling that at last we were on the way to becoming healers of the sick. Sooner or later we became convinced that we could learn the art of taking a medical history from a patient. Even more important, it dawned upon us that the most seasoned clinicians didn't always reach the right conclusions and were occasionally left barking up the wrong tree by placing undue emphasis upon some chance remark that was not really germane to the patient's problem. While practice and more practice would make us reasonably competent most of the time, none of us would ever master completely the difficult and fascinating art of history taking—the basis upon which at least 85 percent of all diagnoses are made.

Our first attempts at physical diagnosis were even more awkward. Since we had no experience upon which to base comparisons, we learned painfully slowly what heart sounds were normal, how big a normal liver was, and where its lower edge could be felt. How loud should breath sounds be when the stethoscope is placed over the shoulder blade? How brisk should a normal knee jerk be, and how hard should the rubber hammer strike the knee? With time one can learn to perform a reasonably complete physical examination in something less than half an hour. Our first attempts lasted half a day or more.

Along the way most of us diagnosed ourselves as having at least one fatal disease. A cough lasting more than twenty-four hours surely signified tuberculosis which would require us to spend a year or two in a sanatorium high on a lonely Alp. Most of us suffered imaginary heart attacks when all we really had was indigestion.

By the time we left the laboratories for the hospital wards, we were fairly sure that we would not flunk out of medical school. This was very reassuring, and I believe none of us had expected to be as free as we were from this particular anxiety. But the pressure to excel was very intense, and the competition very keen because after medical school would come internship, and we all believed that the best students would get the best internships. Actually, we had little to worry about because there were many more good internships than there were medical graduates to fill them. But this we only discovered later.

It was soon apparent that more than good study habits were now required. The more studious drones among us no longer automatically led the pack. Some students with relatively mediocre track records in bacteriology and chemistry turned out to be most at ease with patients and extremely adept at finding out what was wrong with them. One of our most brilliant classmates, who had been in the top 5 percent in every one of our basic science courses, never did master the art of dealing with patients, and not long after graduation we heard he had committed suicide.

As we progressed from one medical specialty to another, we felt very much like blind children learning about an elephant by feeling first one part and then another. "An elephant is like a rope," said one child, grasping the tail. "No, it's like the flap of a tent," said another, holding onto an ear. "No, it's like a telephone pole," said a third, with his arms around a leg, and so on. We began to see that none of us would ever become the "Complete Physician," able to master all phases of medicine and able to treat anybody. We saw this all the more clearly because all of our teachers fervently believed it to be true.

Inhabitants of the ivory towers were deaf to the cries of patients lamenting the disappearance of the family doctor. The general practitioner was held to be the lowest form of medical life. Specialization was not only the best way to go, it was the only way to go. The nearest thing to a general practitioner was an internist, who wouldn't dream of caring for children, delivering babies, or sewing up the simplest little cut in the skin. That few of us thought to question our teachers in this respect is reflected in the fact that more than 90 percent of us became specialists of one kind or another.

In addition to the fact that we were not interested in becoming the sort of physicians our patients were looking for, the push for an early decision as to what specialty to enter had another serious drawback. In order to obtain an internship in the desired specialty, we had to decide which field to enter when we were only halfway through the clinical part of our medical school experience. It was obvious that we could not all be exposed to medicine first, pediatrics next, and so on. The result was that some of us who would have made good surgeons didn't see the inside of an operating room until late in the senior year, long after the die had been cast as far as our choice of medical career was concerned. The only acceptable defense against inability to make up one's mind was to take a rotating internship, but these were fast losing favor in the 1950s, and all but disappeared from the face of the earth in the ensuing decade. Anyone honest enough to admit that he couldn't make up his mind until he had seen more of the possible areas of specialization was labeled indecisive, a quality no less reprehensible in a physician than in a politician.

Deciding upon a specialty was largely a process of elimination. Psychiatry was the first to fall. Although I realized the great need for emotional healing, my exposure to psychiatry in medical school convinced me that I was not cut out to be a psychiatrist. Every Tuesday afternoon we spent an hour talking to a patient, guided by a psychiatrist who oversaw six of us. In the succeeding hour she had us each briefly relate what we had discussed with our patient and suggested areas to explore in the next session a week later. Every Tuesday we saw the same patient and discussed him with the same psychiatrist. Every Thursday we did the same thing, except that on Thursday we had a different patient and a different teacher. At the end of the course one of the teachers gave me an "A" and the other gave me a "D." Deciding that there was a message in there somewhere, I eliminated psychiatry from my list of choices, a decision I have never regretted, although through the years I have always felt that I understood psychiatrists better than many of my surgical colleagues did.

Next to go was dermatology. The idea of caring for people, none of whom died and none of whom ever got well, didn't appeal to the altruism in us. Despite the fact that diagnosis and treatment of skin diseases is in many ways a fascinating and rewarding specialty, not a single one of my classmates became a dermatologist.

The big decision was between medicine and surgery. Either you operated or you didn't. The operators were surgeons, orthopedists, neurosurgeons, obstetricians, etc. The non-operators were internists, pediatricians, psychiatrists, and the like. Because of the way the medical curriculum was designed, I decided I was a non-operator before I had ever participated in an operation. One advantage of being a non-operator was that the internship and residency programs are much shorter than those in the surgical specialties. Having a wife and three children by the time I graduated from medical school, I viewed this as a huge advantage.

Perhaps it was because I was familiar with babies. Perhaps it was because deterioration, decay, and the inherent hopelessness of old age depressed me. Perhaps it was because, being married to one, I wasn't afraid of mothers. Whatever the factors were, I knew that I preferred caring for children to caring for adults. I was sure of this by the end of the third year of medical school, and nothing that has happened to me since has made me change my mind. For me, the only thing that could come close to child care is obstetrics, which I have always felt would have been my second choice. Just as I now hate to relinquish the care of teenagers when they "outgrow" me, I would have hated to turn over to someone else the care of the babies I delivered.

My determination to become a pediatrician was enhanced by a fortunate accident. While I was assigned as a medical student to the pediatric ward, two of the pediatric interns came down with hepatitis. The Chief of Pediatrics invited the first two medical students he encountered to become substitute interns, and I was fortunate enough to be the first to cross his path. An intern is vastly superior to a medical student, not only in the opportunity to see and learn, but also to be noticed. The very best way to get a good recommendation for an internship is to impress the staff with a good performance as a substitute intern. Fortunately, the real interns recovered before I had made any lethal mistakes and the chief sent off a glowing letter about me to the Chairman of the Pediatric Department at Bellevue, where I was accepted without hesitation. The fact that a square peg was being fitted to a round hole did not become apparent for almost two years.

2

Bellevue

Bellevue was the hub of the New York City hospital system, affiliated with Columbia, Cornell, and New York universities. It was considered a great place for training in any specialty because there were no private patients. To neophyte interns private patients were an anathema because their personal physicians made all the important decisions and the interns functioned more or less as errand boys. After two years of watching others take care of patients we were eager for a chance to do it ourselves without further interference.

A week after graduation from medical school the new Bellevue interns were issued the traditional white suits and herded into an auditorium for a briefing on our new duties. There were eighteen pediatric interns, a small group compared to the veritable army of future internists and surgeons. I remember thinking, "Many hands make light work."

All of us expected to work hard, but I think most of us were not prepared for the avalanche of work that descended on us. In my first twenty-four hours I took the histories, did physical examinations, blood counts, urinalyses, and wrote admission orders for thirteen infants, an undertaking which only a short time before would have consumed the better part of a week. The hospital served a large population newly arrived from Puerto Rico, which made history taking a frustrating experience for doctor and parents alike. One brave Puerto Rican mother who spoke a smattering of English, after seeing her own baby safely to bed, stayed with me all night long and helped me grope my way through the admission procedures of five more. Two of the babies I admitted that first night died, one of overwhelming diarrhea and the other of rat bites.

Bellevue was a do-it-yourself place. Blood counts and urinalyses were all done by the interns. The nurses were so few that we did many of the nursing procedures ourselves. We could get anything we needed for our patients as long as we were willing to go and get it. We didn't send specimens to the lab, we took them, and often ran the tests ourselves. We could get x-rays any time we wanted them, as long as we took the patients to the X-ray Department and waited with them until the x-rays were done. The nurses and aides were far too busy to leave the wards.

One of the babies I admitted on the afternoon of my first day appeared only moderately ill at first, but as the night wore on her respirations became more labored and her fever climbed relentlessly. At 11 P.M. a lone student nurse took over the ward of forty-three babies. She immediately recognized how gravely ill this infant was and how helpless I was to do anything about it. The next morning I was congratulated for having shown good judgment in changing the baby's medication in the middle of the night. The little student nurse who had suggested the change was transferred to another ward, or perhaps even to another hospital. I never saw her again, and to this day she remains ignorant of the gratitude I still feel for her. The baby made a rapid and complete recovery.

Although we were left pretty much to sink or swim by ourselves at night, we were exposed to some of the country's most gifted teachers during the day. Among them were Dr. Edith Lincoln, the foremost expert on childhood tuberculosis, and Dr. May Wilson, who knew all there was to know about rheumatic fever. These two diseases, which filled whole wards of forty or fifty beds, have now virtually vanished, though the lessons we learned about heart and lung disease from these two great teachers are as valuable today as they were when we learned them in the early 1950s.

Rheumatic fever tended to recur over and over in children who were susceptible to it. Each attack carried the risk of further damage to the heart valves, and we cared for many children who had been reduced by repeated attacks to a permanent bed-and-chair existence. The most bizarre aspect of rheumatic fever was its effect on the nervous system. St. Vitus' dance, as it was called, was horrible to see. The children were so irritable that at the accidental slamming of a door they would jump almost out of their skins. Their speech was so slurred as to be almost unintelligible, and they had such gross tremors that their handwriting was illegible. The most severely affected could not even hold a pencil.

The first attack of rheumatic fever rarely caused very serious permanent damage, but a mother had only to look around her at the other children on the ward to see what devastation lay in store for her child if recurrences were not prevented. It was known that streptococcal infections caused rheumatic fever and that either penicillin or sulfanilamide, given once a day, would prevent almost all recurrent attacks. It has always seemed inconceivable to me that parents who had seen the ravages of repeated attacks of rheumatic fever would fail to give their child a single tablet once a day, but studies repeatedly showed that more than three fourths abandoned this simple prophylactic measure before the end of the first year. As Sir William Osler said, "It must needs be that offences of this kind come; expect them, and do not be vexed."

The treatment of tuberculosis was based on giving the child every opportunity to overcome the infection by himself. Every form of exertion was forbidden, including walking to the bathroom. The children were kept in the hospital because parents could not be expected to enforce this onerous inactivity day after day and because many of the children would not get good nutrition at home. Their progress was measured by such clinical parameters as cough, fever, and weight loss, and by weekly chest x-rays. At the weekly tuberculosis rounds every chest x-ray each child had ever had was reviewed. We spent hours preparing for these conferences, making sure that the many x-rays were in order. It was not unusual to review forty chest x-rays of a single child. Just as one area of a child's chest would appear to have cleared up completely, Dr. Lincoln would spot a new shadow, so faint that even after she pointed it out to us we often could not be sure it was there. In two or three weeks, subsequent films invariably proved that she had been right.

The *sine qua non* of successful arrest of tuberculosis was three consecutive negative cultures of gastric juice. To obtain these we arrived on the ward early in the morning and passed a long rubber tube into the child's stomach. The small amount of gastric juice we removed from the stomach contained tubercle bacilli which the child had coughed up and swallowed during the night. These hardy organisms withstood the corrosive action of acid stomach juice and multiplied when cultured in the laboratory. As long as the cultures were positive the disease was active, and the child could not be allowed out of bed. When three successive cultures were negative there would be ice cream and cake and a tearful farewell. Nearly all the children cried lustily on leaving the nurses who had grown more dear to them than their own parents during their long confinement.

One group of children whose lives were affected by tuberculosis were the babies born of mothers who had the disease. The tuberculosis organism is not carried across the placenta, so that the babies never had the disease at birth, but if left with their mothers after birth they soon contracted it. We had a whole ward full of babies with nothing wrong with them, growing in the sterile environment of a nursery for weeks or months until their mothers were declared safe to take them home.

From the day I started at Bellevue until I left for Boston a year later I never examined or cared for a single adult. Meanwhile, my ex-classmates who were interns in medicine or surgery never treated a single child. The contrast in our experiences was brought home to me on the day we took the National Board exam. The test consisted of a practical demonstration of our ability to diagnose and treat simple medical and surgical problems. The pediatric portion entailed being sent into a room with four cribs, each containing a baby or young child. At the foot of each crib was a small white card with clues as to the nature of the problem. Three of the problems were obvious and the treatment straightforward, at least to those of us who were interning in pediatrics. The fourth patient was a one-month-old baby whose card said simply "MOTHER HAS TUBERCULOSIS." For pediatric interns from Bellevue this was duck soup. We merely had to tell the examiner that the baby was normal and answer a few questions about normal growth and development, such as when the baby could be expected to sit, stand, and walk. With barely

suppressed glee I watched three surgical interns turn that poor
baby almost inside out trying to find some abnormality that
wasn't there. I was not privileged to hear them tell the examiner
what diseases they had diagnosed, but I'm sure he enjoyed himself hugely at their expense.

While most of the children with tuberculosis appeared completely healthy and their disease was only detected because of
compulsory skin testing, a few were very sick, and two of those
I looked after died. The saddest little boy I ever saw in my life I
saw on the tuberculosis ward at Bellevue. At the end of visiting
hours his mother had departed, leaving him a banana she had
brought from home. He sat in his crib in total silence with tears
streaming down his face because he was too weak to peel it.
When I took it and broke the skin for him his tear-drenched
face lit up with a most radiant smile, and he hugged me with his
tiny arms before turning full attention to his little feast.

Both rheumatic fever and tuberculosis still occur, but fortunately modern antibiotic treatment has made them almost medical curiosities, and many of today's interns have never seen a
child with either disease.

Bellevue was much better known for medical care and teaching than for research, but a surprising amount of clinical research was done there nonetheless. For years the progress of premature babies everywhere was plotted on graphs prepared at
Bellevue. These graphs have a series of curves depicting the optimal weight gain for babies with different birth weights. Babies
who weigh less at birth gain more slowly than those who are
heavier to start with, and it is important to know what can be
expected of any given infant. If they fail to keep up with their
predicted weight gain, they usually have a medical problem
which can often be identified and hopefully corrected. Attempting to force a baby to gain faster than the Bellevue standard indicates is fraught with danger because the tiny infants are prone to
vomit and inhale the excess formula they do not need and cannot
assimilate.

The care of premature babies had been improving rapidly.
Many babies weighing less than three pounds were surviving,
and occasionally an infant who had weighed less than two pounds
at birth would leave the nursery alive. Survival of tiny premature

infants was not without its problems, however. A significant number were found later to be almost totally blind. In an effort to understand this phenomenon every premature baby at Bellevue was examined weekly by an ophthalmologist. The eyes were invariably normal at birth, but soon thereafter the ophthalmologist could see evidence of inflammation behind the lens of the eye. This inflammation was followed by the formation of dense fibrous scar tissue, hence the name of the condition, retrolental fibroplasia.

The cause of retrolental fibroplasia was unknown, and every aspect of the babies' care was scrutinized looking for clues. Someone got the notion that the disease might be caused by keeping the babies in an atmosphere artificially enriched with oxygen longer than was necessary. Bellevue cooperated with a number of other hospitals to test this theory. A randomized card was drawn for every infant on admission to the premature nursery. Those in one group received supplemental oxygen only if they clearly needed it. Those in the other group were kept in an oxygen-enriched atmosphere for seventy-two hours after the need for extra oxygen appeared to have ended. The idea that oxygen, the very essence of life, could be harmful to our tiny infants seemed ridiculous to us, and we considered the whole project a huge waste of time. Toward the end of my stay at Bellevue the code was broken, and it was shown beyond a shadow of a doubt that the primary cause of retrolental fibroplasia *was* oxygen given to tiny infants for a longer time and in higher concentrations than needed. This simple experiment has saved the eyesight of countless premature babies.

In the afternoons we worked in the clinics, to which came hoards of children with all sorts of problems, great and small. They were met by a single nurse who sorted them out according to disease and severity and sent them to one of a dozen different pediatric clinics. This formidable exercise in triage was facilitated by her modest knowledge of Spanish and her phenomenal memory for faces and past complaints. I spent an afternoon with her in the mistaken belief that a doctor could make better sorting decisions than a nurse. After two hundred patients had flashed by I found that I had agreed with her 198 times. In both instances in which I had disagreed she turned out to be right. Eight years later I returned to Bellevue for a brief visit and found her still at her little triage desk, directing the flow of traffic with her uncanny tact and skill.

Among those who helped us most in the clinics were the social workers. The social problems of poverty, broken homes, language barriers, and ignorance were staggering. The resources available to these gallant workers were scant indeed, but they opened my eyes to what could be accomplished by people who knew how the system worked and who cared desperately about their little charges.

Pediatricians who abandon pediatrics and switch to caring for adults rarely do so because of inability to get along with children. It's their lack of rapport with mothers that ultimately does them in. Bellevue was a wonderful place to get to know and like mothers. Despite my difficulties with Spanish, which persisted for all the time I was there, I was greatly attracted to the hundreds of gentle, loving, Puerto Rican mothers I came to know there. I can count the Puerto Rican fathers I knew on the fingers of one hand. They left the rearing of children strictly to their wives, and even when their children grew desperately ill, generally left the mothers to cope all by themselves. Some of their neglect was not entirely benign. The little mother whose baby died from rat bites on my first night at Bellevue returned the next day covered with welts and bruises resulting from her husband's rage when he was confronted with the news of his baby's death.

Shortly after we arrived we started a new tradition. One of the more adventurous members of our intern group persuaded the distributor of Miller Beer to donate two cases of ice cold beer with which to liven up our Friday afternoon conference. There were so many of us that nobody got more than one or, at the most, two cans, but it did our morale a world of good to know that ours was the only service in the hospital to be so favored. Our Chief, Dr. Holt, stopped in for a moment on his way home, gently declined the beer which was proffered to him, and took his leave as soon as he saw that all was well. The next week we called the distributors of Schlitz and informed them that last week the Miller people had sent down two cases of cold beer for the doctors who cared for the sick children at Bellevue. They promptly volunteered to do the same, and the pattern was established. Thereafter, no distributor refused us, and week after week we were able to publish a notice that on Friday afternoon at 4 P.M. we would hold a conference at which there would be "two cases." Dr. Holt always came, never accepted a beer, which he felt had been donated for our enjoyment, and never stayed more than a few minutes to dampen our fun. He always brought his hat and coat, and so far as I can remember, never failed to wear a pair of rubbers no matter how brightly the sun might be shining.

Despite the fact that Dr. Holt was widely respected as one of the foremost pediatric teachers of his day, he was the most unpretentious of men. He conducted rounds in the gentlest manner, never displaying disappointment or anger when we recounted our inept therapeutic failures. The senior residents, who had more direct contact with him than we interns did, revered him.

Dr. Holt was a world authority on infant nutrition and had devoted years to improving infant formulas, a fact we acknowledged at our Christmas party. Everyone drew a name from a hat. The object was to buy a Christmas present costing no more than twenty-five cents for the individual whose name we had drawn. The intern who drew Dr. Holt's name got him a forty-quart milk can with a half pint of milk in it so that Dr. Holt could have fun adding things to it.

The Director of Pediatric Clinics was Dr. Saul Krugman, whose textbook on pediatric infections was to become a classic. He was, like Dr. Holt, a man of great humility. His devotion to the interns knew no bounds, and he was always ready to drop his formidable workload to come with us to examine a patient and help us prescribe properly for him. We found his lectures somewhat dry and dull due to his flat delivery, but later when his book was published, we recognized what gems those lectures had been as we read chapter after chapter knowing at every turn of the page what he would say next.

Our most gifted teacher was Dr. Edwin Pratt, who later became Chairman of the Department of Pediatrics at the University of Cincinnati. His areas of expertise were endocrinology, especially diabetes, of which we saw a surprising amount in children, and intravenous therapy which many, many children needed. The margin for error in tiny infants was very small, and most of us approached the giving of intravenous fluids to babies with great insecurity until he taught us how much sodium and potassium to add to the bottles we hung above our little patients.

One morning I presented to Dr. Pratt the case of a baby who had died during the night. As he listened to my story I could tell that he was perplexed. When I finished he asked me, "What did the chest x-ray show?" I replied that I had felt the baby was too sick to go to the X-ray Department, so I had not ordered one. "Well, you might be right," he said, "but I doubt it. Just remember, the sicker they are, the more important it is to find out what is the matter with them." This penetrating observation, made so gently on that morning many years ago, was the most important lesson I learned at Bellevue, or indeed in any of my later training. All of my subsequent experience has confirmed the fundamental importance of establishing a diagnosis before beginning to treat a patient. All good physicians do this; all great teachers advise it in one way or another, but I never heard the principle expressed more succinctly.

The year I spent at Bellevue was a happy and rewarding one, and I was urged to stay on when it was over. Had I done so my professional life would have been very different than it turned out to be, for at Bellevue I saw very little surgery, and what I saw did little to incline me toward becoming a surgeon. So inept were the surgeons at dealing with children that one to whom I sent a child to have a cut finger sutured sent him back to me with a note indicating that the child refused to be sewn up. I turned the note over and wrote on the back, "Children protest, but they never refuse." An hour later the child returned with his laceration neatly sutured.

The trouble with Bellevue was that it was in the middle of New York City. While I was on duty at the hospital thirty-six out of forty-eight hours Patty was raising three children in an apartment on the fourteenth floor. The urge to move to a more rural setting was irresistible, and when an opening at the Boston Children's Hospital arose I snatched it eagerly, unaware of how the move would change my future.

3

On to Boston

When I began to work there in 1954, the Boston Children's Hospital was considered by many to be the best children's hospital in the world. True, the closer one was to Boston, the firmer was the conviction, but in many ways it did live up to its venerable reputation. At about three hundred beds, it was just the right size. It was large enough to have talent in depth and small enough to foster a genuine camaraderie among physicians working in the many different disciplines of child care. At a time when many children's hospitals were getting by with the part-time services of a single neurosurgeon, the Boston Children's Hospital had two who worked there only, and the same was true in most of the other surgical and medical divisions. The hospital was able to provide a uniformity of superb medical care which smaller institutions could admire but could not duplicate.

Talented people came to Boston and tended to stay there because of a feeling that there was no place else to move up to. Harvard was the premier medical school in the days before government subsidy. The only reasons for leaving the Boston Children's Hospital were a hankering to live in another part of the country or the opportunity to leave a junior position from which promotion was blocked by older people who might stay on forever. Nearly every one who left was offered a more senior position elsewhere, often the chance to head a department at a very young age.

The fortunate combination of size and prestige attracted a superb group of house officers, the interns and residents who contributed greatly to making the place run. At a time when many smaller children's hospitals were struggling to fill their quotas of physicians in training, the Boston Children's had long waiting lists. The house officers who rose to the top in medicine and surgery at Boston Children's truly were the cream of the crop. When I arrived in Boston, as when I had started medical school, I was filled with wonder that I had been fortunate enough to be included.

Perhaps the greatest attraction of all was the caliber of the senior staff. It is fair to say that no group of pediatric specialists anywhere in the world were contributing more to advancing the forefront of child care. To work for a time under the tutelage of one of these giants and to come in some measure under the influence of all of them was the ultimate lure to the Boston Children's Hospital.

For Patty and me, with our three small children, Boston offered one more inducement, a chance to live in the country. A ten-minute drive from the hospital brought us to a large country estate where we lived in an apartment on the second floor of a barn. I suppose we would be surprised now to see how small it really was, but coming from a two-room apartment fourteen floors above the pavement of Manhattan, we found our new home spacious and luxurious. In addition to a flock of children, our immediate predecessors had happily raised a litter of Irish Setter puppies in this barn apartment. Wunderbar, our little Dachshund, was in seventh heaven.

As the summer wore on we discovered two problems with the barn. The building swayed in the wind like the mast of a tall ship. It was dependent for heat on an antiquated coal furnace tended sporadically by an ancient caretaker with a penchant for lengthy and unpredictable absences. Patty became expert at stoking the furnace—it was infinitely easier to keep going than to rekindle. She soon discovered that no matter what she did at bedtime, the monster simply would not keep going all night without attention, a feature made worse by the fact that the furnace could be approached only by going down a steep unlighted stairway outside the building.

At the hospital my first exposure to formal teaching was a Saturday morning conference conducted by Sidney Gellis. Dr. Gellis was, among other things, an expert on jaundice in children, but his interests covered the whole range of children's illnesses, and he could hold his own in debates with all of the surgical specialists. His conferences always began with a quiz at which he showed us a photograph or x-ray of a child with features typical of a specific illness. The first unknown he presented I thought absurdly simple, and I was amazed when no one offered a diagnosis. I had seen at least a hundred similar x-rays at Bellevue, and finally ventured to volunteer that the child had rickets. I was the hero of the moment and my reward was the assignment to prepare a ten-minute lecture to the group the following Saturday on any topic I chose. Not wanting to risk talking about anything with which I was the least bit unfamiliar, I chose atlanto-axial subluxation, and discovered to my delight that it was one of the few conditions with which Dr. Gellis was totally unfamiliar. During my very last week at Bellevue the Chief of Orthopedics had described this condition in which the two highest vertebrae in the neck become partially dislocated. Typically, the child has an inflammation of the throat, which is thought by some to impart a certain laxity to the ligaments holding these two vertebrae in line. The child, often in a deep sleep at night, allows his head to flop to one side for a time, and upon awakening has a stiff neck which causes extreme pain when he attempts to turn his head. Simple traction and a brief period of relaxation allow the vertebrae to slip back into alignment and the pain miraculously disappears. All sorts of painful and ineffective measures are apt to be carried out by those not familiar with the condition. The article to which we had been referred contained a simple diagram which I was able to copy in a large chalk drawing on the blackboard. It was an absurdly simple presentation, but it caught Dr. Gellis' imagination, a fact that was to be of inestimable help to me a few years later. Oddly enough, a few weeks later my daughter Kate developed the condition and was promptly cured by a gentle x-ray technician who soothingly relaxed her on the x-ray table and repositioned the vertebrae while attempting to straighten her head for an x-ray. Kate walked out of the x-ray room as normal as pie to the astonishment of the orthopedist who had ordered her admission to the hospital where he had predicted she would have to stay for a week to ten days.

As it had been at Bellevue, my first assignment in Boston was to the baby ward, where I soon found out that life here was going to be different. Very few of the babies came from around the corner; a few of them had come halfway around the world. Very few had the common problems with which I was familiar, such as diarrhea or malnutrition. Nearly all had been referred because conventional methods in outlying hospitals had failed to solve their problems, and many had problems for which solutions were unknown. The abundance of nursing help was astonishing to me. When an intravenous infusion was to be started everything was in readiness and all I had to do was hold the needle still while the nurse threaded the baby onto it. Only the most critically ill had to be accompanied by a doctor to the X-ray Department, and invariably a nurse went with him. We did have to draw blood samples for the laboratory, but once they were drawn we simply handed them to a nurse who saw to all the details of labeling them, filling out the requisition forms, and recording the results in the chart. The results returned with an alacrity that at Bellevue would have been unthinkable. The nurses were full of helpful suggestions which my early experience with the little student nurse at Bellevue had taught me to heed. I've always wondered why so many doctors are reluctant to take suggestions from nurses. It seems that the more obstinately they refuse to accept advice, the more desperately they need it. An insecure ego can be a physician's own worst enemy.

The self-reliance that had been imparted to me at Bellevue was a great asset, and I was able to compete with my fellows in getting the basic chores done with dispatch, leaving time to take advantage of the many conferences and teaching sessions. There were plenty of these on medical subjects, and we were kept informed of them by a daily mimeographed schedule given out by the chief medical resident. I soon discovered that there were a lot of things going on in other departments as well, and that the best way to find out about them was to sit in the house officers' lounge late in the evenings when I was on duty at night. Promptly at 11 P.M. the door would open and in would come a basket loaded with bread, peanut butter, jelly, and fruit; mainly bananas. Members of all the services descended on this basket like locusts and in fifteen minutes only crusts of bread were left, but in these fifteen minutes one could find out what our colleagues in surgery, neurosurgery, orthopedics, pathology, and radiology were doing while we tended our medical charges. I soon found out that the field of child care was much wider than I had previously supposed, and was swept up in the enthusiasm of people pursuing lives different from my own. Often, alerted by what I had heard during these peanut-butter-and-jelly sessions, I was able to watch operations in the middle of the night.

The operating rooms at the Children's Hospital were small and very old-fashioned. Two of them had galleries that could accommodate about a dozen observers. The galleries were a floor above the operating rooms and consisted of two benches opposite each other separated by slanting glass partitions, which looked like a transparent chicken coop suspended above the operating table. The center of the top was open so that by raising his voice the surgeon could tell us what he was doing. If he stood aside, we could gaze right down into the wound, though heads and shoulders blocked our view much of the time. It was in one of these rooms that Dr. Robert Gross, the premier pediatric surgeon of the day, had first successfully ligated a patent ductus arteriosus and thus opened up the whole field of cardiac surgery. In this same room a few years later he had first successfully removed a coarctation of the aorta for which he had barely missed being awarded the Nobel Prize. None of the cardiovascular surgery went on at night of course, but I was able to watch appendectomies and other emergency general surgery as well as occasional neurosurgical and orthopedic procedures. The excitement of these midnight ventures into the surgical gallery made some of our routine medical care seem even more routine than it actually was.

After my tour on the infant ward I was assigned to the emergency room, where I found things much less exciting than I had at Bellevue. The pace was much slower and the help so abundant that the relatively few patients could be handled with dispatch. Since I knew I would eventually be going on the cardiac ward, I took advantage of an offer from Ricardo Abbugadas to spend my spare moments with him learning to read electrocardiograms.

These were assembled in a small laboratory deep in the basement of the hospital where we were totally isolated from the outside world. Ricardo was from Argentina and was spending a year of fellowship in cardiology in Boston. He was fascinated by America, which he was seeing for the first time. I learned far more from him about Boston and its environs than about elec-trocardiograms, which to this day I find very confusing.

One afternoon I spent several hours with Ricardo in his sub-terranian cubbyhole only to find upon emerging that New En-gland had been ravaged by a hurricane. Patty had tried to call me to say that the barn was bending like a reed in the wind, but she was cut off from communication because the telephone lines were down. She had had enough warning to be able to lay in a supply of candles and sterno, her only sources of light and cook-ing heat for the next week. Fortunately, the old coal monster in the basement was not dependent on electricity, as were all the oil burners in the area, and she and the children were relatively comfortable until the roads were finally cleared and contact with the outside world reestablished. I commiserated with Ricardo that he had missed the first hurricane New England had seen in more than fifteen years. "Ah well," said Ricardo, "next hurri-cane." Within three weeks we were treated to a second one.

These two hurricanes coupled with the increasingly frigid midnight dashes down the outside stairs to fuel the furnace con-vinced Patty that we should abandon the barn. We met with a real estate agent who took us through a huge house far beyond our means or needs. He learned enough about us by listening to our comments about this palatial dwelling to suggest a more modest house that he felt would suit us to a "T." We agreed to look at it that very afternoon though we would have to hurry as the sun was setting and the electricity had been turned off. We toured the little house in record time with daylight fast disap-pearing. The agent extolled the location, which was indeed ideal for our purposes, and the bedrooms which were more numerous than we needed but very nice indeed. He whisked us through the kitchen which was primitive by any standard and hastened on to the living room which he felt was the best feature of the house. Patty took one look at the delapidated kitchen with its coal stove and total lack of storage space and declared, "That would be no problem." I don't know who was more surprised, the agent or I. As darkness fell we assured him that we would think about it and get in touch with him.

Two days later our ridiculously low offer was accepted and for $12,500 we became the proud owners of a five-bedroom house on "Pill Hill," about a mile from the Children's Hospital. This astute move, for which Patty must accept full credit, was the beginning of a remarkably successful chain of real estate transactions that enabled us to keep ahead of the inflation which then only a few people saw coming. Maybe she did; I certainly did not.

Our first steps were to cut back a jungle of overgrown bushes, build a narrow driveway, take off an ugly porch, and paint the exterior a dark, battle-ship gray. We had a contractor for the driveway and a carpenter to help with the porch, but we did a good deal of the work ourselves. I was extremely proud of my first house and thought it the most handsome of dwellings. Just as the last of the paint was dry we were visited by a friend from New York who deflated me completely by observing, "Wow, that one looks straight out of Charles Addams, doesn't it?"

On the day we moved in, a cheery face appeared from next door and we were welcomed to the neighborhood by Eleanor Hendren. She and Hardy had recently bought an equally run-down but basically solid house no more than twelve feet from ours and were well ahead of us in renovating it. They became two of our closest friends, and while Hardy and I were off at our respective hospitals for thirty-six of every forty-eight hours, Patty and Eleanor were both father and mother to nine children, four of ours and five of theirs.

Sooner or later each of our own children needed medical care, though fortunately not for anything more serious than sore throats and the like. From the plethora of medical talent most of the doctors chose Dr. William Berenberg. He was so sought after and so generous with the free care he gave physicians' children that we wondered how he was able to make a living. He would discuss at any length we wished the reasons for his recommendations, and our wives were as pleased and grateful for his care as we medical neophytes were. His skill in solving children's problems was legendary. One afternoon I called him for an anxious mother who had brought her little girl to the emergency room with what she believed to be a rapidly growing abdominal tumor. Dr. Berenberg asked a few questions and elicited the fact that the family had hastily retreated from their burning home and that the little girl had refused to use the unfamiliar toilet in the hotel where they were staying.

"What color was the toilet seat in your home?" he asked.

"Why, it was blue," said the startled mother.

"Well then," said Dr. Berenberg, "take her to the ladies room at the Sunset Lounge. They have blue toilets. If that doesn't work call me in half an hour." After instructing us to have a catheterization set ready for him should she return, he left. Fifteen minutes later his nurse called to inform us that the catheter would not be needed. The child had voided an ocean as soon as she had been placed on the blue toilet seat and the abdominal tumor had been flushed happily down the drain.

Very few premature babies were referred long distances to the Boston Children's Hospital. In those days every pediatrician considered himself an expert in the care of prematures, and even the Beth Israel Hospital, which was only a few blocks away, had its own premature nursery. The premature nursery was one of the smallest units in the Boston Children's Hospital, usually containing between six and ten infants. A large number of senior pediatricians shared responsibility for these babies on a rotating basis with the predictable result that nobody considered prematurity a field of primary interest. The unit was held together by an eccentric but fanatically devoted head nurse named Miss Berg. She probably had a first name, but no one seems to remember it. Perhaps because my experience at the much larger premature nursery at Bellevue had prepared me better than most of the other house officers, or perhaps just because she was a bit nutty, Miss Berg liked me and together we shared an exciting adventure in her little domain.

About supper time one evening we admitted a tiny baby to the nursery. Although I noticed nothing unusual about him except for his birth weight of just under three pounds, Miss Berg decided at first glance that something was wrong with him. She stayed far into the night, much to the distress of the nurse who had come to relieve her, and before morning had come to the conclusion that the baby was diabetic. Before he was twenty-four hours old she had convinced me to do the appropriate tests, and we found ourselves in charge of a diabetic infant younger and smaller than any that had previously been reported in the medical literature.

The librarian at the Harvard Medical Library could find nothing to guide us in caring for him except for a series of articles by a Doctor Brush who had reported on a small group of older children. These articles correctly predicted that the infant's need for insulin would remain relatively high for a few days and then drop over a period of twelve to fourteen days to a fraction of the original amount. A single cubic centimeter of the most dilute standard insulin preparation contained forty units, about ten times the amount he tolerated during the first week. We diluted this with ten times its weight of sterile water and thus were able to measure fairly accurately an amount of insulin appropriate for his needs. For about ten days the baby flourished, regaining his birth weight in four days and progressing nicely along one of the lines on the Bellevue growth chart indicating a normal rate of gain for a baby of his birth weight. The objective was to give enough insulin to keep all traces of acetone from his urine but not so much as to eliminate a small amount of sugar. We did these simple tests in the nursery. Urine containing acetone turned pink when mixed with the proper reagent, and urine boiled in a pale blue solution turned green with a trace of sugar and coppery red with a large excess. On the eleventh day the blue solution remained blue, indicating that our four units of insulin a day had now become more than the baby needed. By adding a small amount of water each day to the bottle from which we drew the insulin we were able to follow in miniature the table in Dr. Brush's article, gradually reducing the daily intake of insulin. After twelve more days the baby's daily requirements had dropped from four to one and a half units, where it leveled off exactly as the Brush regime had predicted.

Word of this little drama spread throughout the hospital, and I was asked to present the baby's case to the senior staff at the weekly Grand Rounds. Miss Berg and I decided that we had a pretty exciting tale to tell, one that would be even better if we knew the diabetic or prediabetic status of every member of the baby's family.

The whole family, grandparents and all, lived within a few

blocks of the hospital, and bright and early on Sunday morning they all assembled, having eaten nothing since bedtime the night before. We drew fasting blood samples from all of them and then gave them measured amounts of sugar mixed with a little water. This simple syrup tasted awful, but they all downed it without complaint and we drew more blood samples, one, two, and four hours after they had swallowed it. We now had twenty-eight little test tubes of blood, which I carted off to the laboratory only to find that because it was Sunday there was no technician on duty. Fortunately, blood-sugar determinations are relatively easy to run, and by supper time I had seven neat little graphs showing the glucose tolerance curves of the baby's eighteen-month-old brother, father, mother, and all four grandparents. None were frankly diabetic, but one of the grandmothers had a prediabetic curve suggesting that the baby derived a genetic tendency to diabetes from his mother's side of the family.

Public speaking comes easily to me now after twenty years of lecturing to medical students, but as I gazed out over the sea of faces on the day of Grand Rounds that winter morning I had a giant case of stage fright. I finally found my voice, after which a good story, solidly documented, pretty much told itself, and when it was over the staff burst into applause. Applause at these solemn Grand Round sessions was almost as rare as applause in church, and I was so overwhelmed that I very nearly burst into tears.

Three days later the baby developed fulminating diarrhea and died. I vowed then and there never again to recount a therapeutic success in public before the patient had been safely discharged from the hospital.

The baby's mother came to the hospital where I pleaded with her for permission for an autopsy, but the father refused to come. Usually if permission for an autopsy cannot be obtained after an hour of wheedling, it will not be forthcoming, but I persisted and finally, after her husband refused to talk with her even over the telephone, she slammed down the receiver and signed the permission form. The autopsy shed no light either on the diabetes or on the cause for the diarrhea, and in this empty fashion our adventure came to a bitterly disappointing end.

4

Leukemia

The top floor of the hospital's new wing was set aside for children with leukemia. No one went up there if it wasn't absolutely necessary, and we residents all dreaded the day when our assignment to the leukemia ward would begin.

On a bleak, winter morning Joyce McKenna took me on my orientation tour. I think when Florence Nightingale dreamed of the ideal nurse she must have had Joyce in mind. She was by far the youngest head nurse in the hospital, a radiantly beautiful girl who could easily have been mistaken for one of the student nurses, all of whom were five or six years younger than I. As she moved through her crowded ward she radiated confidence and compassion. Everyone felt stronger and braver in her presence, and as I followed her I felt a little of my own terror of leukemia begin to melt away.

Leukemia is by far the commonest form of cancer in children, affecting nearly half of all children who develop malignancy in any form. Despite the best care known in the 1950s most children with leukemia lived only a few weeks. Usually the course was relentlessly downhill, but a few children experienced spectacular remissions, during which all traces of the disease seemed to vanish. After a few weeks of joyous and robust good health it always reappeared. Occasionally, a second remission would occur, but in the end leukemia always prevailed. In 1955 no child anywhere in the world had ever recovered permanently.

The problem lay in the bone marrow where the blood cells are formed. Bone marrow contains millions of blood cells in varying stages of maturity. Normally, only cells that are almost perfectly mature are released from the marrow to circulate in the blood. Of the three types, red cells are the most numerous. Their function is to pick up oxygen in the lungs and transport it throughout the body. The smallest are the platelets, tiny cells without which blood will not clot. The third kind are the white blood cells which are important defenders against infection. Normal marrow is remarkably sensitive, responding within minutes to a need for more blood cells. By noting an increasing number of white cells in the blood one can detect the beginning of an infection hours before most other signs appear. No specific bacteria have ever been implicated as causing leukemia, but the profusion of young white cells in the marrow of leukemic children has tantalized researchers with the notion that somehow the body is trying to respond to an unidentified form of infection.

In some mysterious way leukemia blocks the ability of white cells to mature. Young white cells, too immature to participate in combating infection, jam the marrow and crowd out the precoursers of all other forms. The blood becomes flooded with white cells, giving rise to the name "leukemia" which means "white blood." They are "white" like water rather than like milk, whereas the red cells really are red, so the blood of leukemic children is red like the blood of other children, though often paler than normal.

What triggered the wild and uncontrolled multiplication of young white cells, and what mysterious force prevented them from maturing? Why, when most succumbed within days to the relentless onrush of the disease, did a few children recover for a time? Why did adults handle the disease better than children? In the end, they too invariably died, but adults tended to live for many months, even years, with what seemed to be the same disease that children could withstand only for a few weeks. If this one disease could be conquered, half of all childhood cancer would be wiped out in a single stroke, and perhaps the same discovery could provide the answer for adults with leukemia as well.

Among the scientists caught up in the challenge of leukemia was Dr. Sidney Farber, who dominated the leukemia ward at

Boston Children's Hospital. Sidney Farber and Joyce McKenna were a study in contrasts. She was the essence of warmth and compassion. He was an impeccable block of ice. Stiff and erect in his starched white coat, he seemed to march whenever he walked. He had a tiny black moustache, and at the late night peanut-butter-and-jelly sessions more than one resident had been heard to wonder out loud how many times a day he trimmed it. No one could remember having heard him laugh, or even seen him smile. He kept himself completely aloof from the daily care of children, giving orders but never participating in the slightest way in carrying them out. He never seemed to share our joy when one of the children improved or our grief when they succumbed. Watching him stalk off to his laboratory after his daily rounds was like watching the departure of Napoleon.

How did this vain and lonely man propose to conquer leukemia? Dr. Farber expected no spectacular breakthrough. He viewed himself as a soldier engaged in a war that would last for many years and would be won inch by inch. He was brutally frank in his discussions with parents, but he could and always did hold out the slim hope that theirs might be the first child to make a complete and permanent recovery. It was that hope, which for him was not a hope at all but a firm, unshakable belief, that sustained us all. It made it possible for us to inflict all sorts of painful procedures on these helpless little patients, and for the parents it somehow lessened the agony of watching their precious children slip away from them.

Dr. Farber was convinced that surgery and x-ray therapy, the two most powerful weapons of the day against most other forms of cancer, could not be expected to cure leukemia. Leukemia involved the marrow in every bone of the body. There was no way a surgeon could remove it. A few patients had been subjected to total body irradiation, but the young leukemia cells were so resistant to the x-ray beams that they could be killed only by an amount of x-ray energy that killed all the healthy cells in the marrow too, leaving the children totally powerless to recover. If, after all of the child's own marrow cells had been killed, bone marrow from healthy people was transplanted to them, the transplanted cells never survived.

There had to be a different approach, a medicine that would

specifically attack the leukemia cells, leaving all other living cells at least relatively unharmed. There were very few chemical substances to choose from. Nitrogen mustard was one of them. Even in small amounts, nitrogen mustard is very toxic. If nitrogen mustard were to help leukemic children, the amount given must be critical. Too little, and the malignant cells would recover; too much, and the treatment itself would kill the child. Dr. Farber had made many attempts to find the balance, but had never found it. Perhaps a combination of drugs would be safer and more effective than one alone. It was a slender hope, but Dr. Farber was convinced that it was possible. As he paced the wards, his beady eyes searched for the faintest clue that one of the combinations of drugs we had given on his instruction was eliciting even the slightest favorable response.

Individual white cells survive only a short time after being released from the marrow. A decrease in their number in the blood meant that a few hours earlier their proliferation in the marrow had been slowed. Whether this was due to a strengthening of the child's natural defenses or to the effect of the drugs we were giving was never certain. Only by analyzing thousands of blood counts and relating them to the timing and dosage of the medications could a pattern be discerned. It was a task for which Dr. Farber's aloof and coldly detached personality ideally suited him. After many months and hundreds of trials he had succeeded in extending the average life-span of leukemic children by less than a week. But it *was* longer when his drugs were used than when they were not, and that to him was what really mattered.

Involved as we were in the daily care of the children and the fears and anxieties of the parents, we had little hope of recognizing patterns. It was impossible for us not to be profoundly affected by the intense feelings of these brave mothers and fathers, particularly so because they practically never left their children's bedsides. Visiting hours were all very well in other parts of the hospital where the children were less ill, but when the remaining time to be together was measured in days or even hours banishing the parents was unthinkable.

Joyce did everything in her power to involve the parents in caring for their children. She went far beyond encouraging them to bathe and feed and read storybooks by the hour. Most of the mothers became expert at timing intravenous infusions. This was a tremendous help to us because many of the medications were very irritating to the veins, and if the infusion was allowed to stop for even a few minutes a clot would form at the tip of the needle necessitating removal and insertion of a new one in a different vein. With each passing day, as vein after vein became obstructed, there remained fewer and fewer sites where an infusion could be started successfully.

Involving parents was not without its price because when things went wrong they always blamed themselves, and sometimes their sense of guilt was nearly overwhelming. In addition, it put them in a position to be bitterly critical of any lack of attention on our part. Dr. Farber demanded our complete attention when we went on rounds with him, permitting no distraction no matter how critically we might feel we were needed elsewhere. An infusion ran dry one morning just as we were beginning our rounds, and when I admitted to the mother that because I had been delayed I would have to remove the needle and insert a new one she treated me to a look of loathing that has haunted me for more than twenty years.

At the end of six weeks I was exhausted and emotionally drained. I was tremendously relieved to be leaving behind me the endless suffering and grief and Dr. Farber's almost inhuman coldness. At the same time I felt a deep satisfaction in having fought briefly beside him in the grim war he was convinced would one day be won with chemotherapy.

The passing years have proved him right. Today, half of all leukemic children who were started on modern drug therapy five years ago are alive and apparently perfectly healthy. Other researchers in many lands have extended his concept of chemotherapy to help children and adults with many different forms of cancer, but it all began in the mind of Sidney Farber.

The little girl whose intravenous infusion I had let run dry died during my last night on the leukemia ward. I was convinced that the mother hated me with every fiber of her being, but she thanked me from the bottom of her grief-stricken heart for having tried to help her little girl. Joyce McKenna told me to be sure to come back and visit, but I never did.

Soon after I left the leukemia ward I let a kindly impulse get
me into trouble. Dr. Diamond asked me early one morning to be
on the look-out for a little girl with leukemia who was coming
down from Maine. Dr. Diamond was the Chief of Hematology,
and even though Dr. Farber would be looking after her once the
diagnosis was confirmed, protocol called for one of the hematol-
ogists to check her over first. Knowing that the referring doctor
was an experienced pediatrician, I felt that having Dr. Diamond
confirm his diagnosis would be superfluous. Besides, I had hoped
I never again would have to deal with the family of a leukemic
child. But protocol was protocol.

Night was falling by the time the distraught parents finally arrived, having traveled all day through a driving snow storm.
Their little girl was miserable, obviously sick, and very tired, but
I noticed that she brightened up considerably after wolfing
down a very generous supper. I knew that the parents had left
home before breakfast and had been afraid to stop even for a
snack because of the storm, but still I felt the child's appetite distinctly unusual. Even Joyce McKenna could rarely coax a child
with leukemia to eat so eagerly.

Her doctor had suspected leukemia with good reason. Her
body was covered with painless little bruises. The parents could
give no history of an accident, and the child was so outgoing and
friendly that I was sure she had not been abused. Bruises like hers
can simply appear without provocation whenever the bone marrow falls behind in the job of producing platelets, the tiny color-
less cells that are essential to normal blood clotting. I knew there
were other diseases that could cause this marrow disfunction, but
every child I had ever seen with bruises like these had had leukemia.

I drew the blood samples and stained the smears as Dr. Diamond had ordered. Sure enough, her blood was almost totally
devoid of platelets, but to my surprise I could find no abnormal
white blood cells at all. It seemed only kind to allay the parents'
fears, and I brashly announced that I did not think their little girl
had leukemia.

I raced off to find Dr. Diamond, but in allowing the little girl
to eat supper I had wasted so much time that he had left for a
speaking engagement and could not be reached until morning.

The parents went off to find lodging for the night, blessing me profusely for easing their minds. As I watched them kiss their little girl good night a cold wave of anxiety swept over me. What if I was wrong? What if she did have leukemia after all? I ached to warn them that I might be mistaken, that they should wait to talk to Dr. Diamond in the morning, but their joy was so compelling that I bit my tongue and said nothing.

I was in Dr. Diamond's office at seven-thirty in the morning, desperately hoping he could resolve the problem at once, but he wasn't there. On his desk was a crowded schedule beginning with a lecture to some forty medical students at eight, rounds with a group of foreign visitors at nine, and meetings until midafternoon. Unless by some miracle he came in early, he wouldn't get to look at my blood smears until at least three o'clock.

The little clock on his desk ticked off the minutes with exasperating lethargy until at two minutes of eight he dashed in, scooped up his lecture notes and departed without so much as a nod in my direction.

It was to be one of the longest days of my life. The foreign visitors arrived before he had finished his lecture and occupied his every minute. Meeting merged with meeting without so much as a moment in between. The hospital routine went on as if nothing had happened. Nobody seemed to care that the parents of a beautiful little girl were waiting to hear from the final authority that she was not doomed to die. I went through my duties in a daze. It was as if I were no longer a doctor but had been transformed by my indiscretion into a parent. I saw the hospital as parents must see it; a cold and heartless place where teaching, meetings, even lunch were more important than concern for their child.

Finally, about four o'clock, Dr. Diamond turned his attention to the microscope. As he scanned the slides his concentration was absolute. It was as if he were surrounded by a giant glass dome. Gone were the medical students. Gone were the visitors from London and Paris. The matters he had discussed in the endless series of meetings were entirely cast aside. I could have been a million miles away.

At long last, with his perpetual scowl masking whatever he

might be thinking, he told me to summon the parents. As I listened to him explain to them that their little girl did not have leukemia but a benign disease called thrombocytopenic purpura from which she would almost certainly recover without any treatment whatever, I felt my heart pounding as if I had run a marathon. Whether or not he noticed that the parents didn't seem surprised to hear what he told them I'll never know. But I'll always wonder.

5

Rh Babies

In December I was sent down the street to spend six weeks in the newborn nursery at the Boston Lying-In Hospital. Devoted entirely to obstetrics and gynecology, this hospital was a happy and peaceful place in which to work. The corridors were filled with proud new fathers and the nurseries with contented, healthy babies. The atmosphere was placid and serene. After a heavy dose of illness and anxiety I found it a wonderful relief to spend some time in a place where every new baby was expected to be normal, and the great majority were. Obstetrics is hard work, the hours long and unpredictable, but it was easy to see why obstetricians love their profession. Nothing erases weariness like the look on a mother's face when she sees her new baby for the first time.

The fact that things nearly always turned out happily made the rare tragedies appear all the more stark. One night I rushed a newborn baby to the operating room at Children's Hospital where the surgeon tried in vain to close a huge hole in the baby's diaphragm. Because the defect had allowed the baby's stomach and part of his liver to slip up into the chest several weeks before birth, his lungs had not had space enough in which to develop normally. Despite an operation of utmost delicacy, the baby simply could not take in enough air to stay alive. It's hard enough to explain a child's death under any circumstances, but there just didn't seem to be any answer at all when the parents of this newborn baby asked me, "Why?"

Occasionally, after what seemed to be a perfectly normal pregnancy and delivery, we would watch a baby slowly develop signs of respiratory distress. As the hours went by his breathing would grow more and more labored and his healthy pink color would turn to an ashen grayish blue. On his tiny chest x-ray we could see that a diffuse haziness involved every part of his lungs. Oxygen helped for a time, and occasionally, after two or three days, the effort of breathing subsided and the baby went on to recover completely. More often, however, even when we turned the oxygen up to 100 percent, the baby eventually tired and died. At autopsy we could see a clear pink membrane resembling rose-tinted glass lining the air passages in the lungs. We knew nothing to do for babies with hyaline membrane disease, as it is called, except to give them oxygen and hope for the best. Things were pretty much the same ten years later when hyaline membrane disease snuffed out the life of President and Mrs. Kennedy's baby.

Pediatricians at Boston Children's and obstetricians at the Lying-In Hospital worked closely together on a number of projects. Among the most exciting of these was unraveling the mysteries of the Rh factor, for which much credit goes to Dr. Diamond's associate, Dr. Frederick Allen.

A great many babies begin to turn faintly yellow when they are two or three days old, so many in fact that this mild jaundice, which lasts about a week, is considered a normal phase of development. But we saw a few babies who began to turn yellow an hour or two after birth, and by the time they were twenty-four hours old were deeply stained from head to toe. Many of them died, and those who recovered were often severely retarded, with spastic limbs and stiff necks and backs. The jaundice cleared, but the damage to the nervous system was profound and permanent.

Virtually always these babies had older brothers or sisters who were perfectly normal, but once a mother had given birth to one baby with this severe jaundice her subsequent babies were usually also affected, and the process tended to grow more severe with each succeeding child. It was not uncommon for a mother, after giving birth to one or two perfectly normal infants, to go through half a dozen pregnancies without ever again taking a living baby home from the hospital. The disorder seemed especially frequent among Catholics, not because of ethnic or religious factors, but because Catholics tended to have large families.

The pigment producing the yellow color is bilirubin which is formed whenever red blood cells are destroyed. An unusually rapid destruction of red cells normally occurs soon after birth when the baby stops taking in oxygen via the placenta and begins to use his lungs. With the lungs functioning normally a baby needs only about three fourths as many red cells as he needed before birth. During the few days required to break down the extra cells the liver often falls behind in the job of removing bilirubin from the blood, and the skin turns faintly yellow. Once the extra red cells have been eliminated the destruction slows, the liver catches up, and the jaundice disappears. Meanwhile, the bone marrow appears to respond to a signal that there are plenty of red cells in the circulation and production of new red blood cells temporarily comes to a halt.

The sick babies behaved differently. The destruction of red cells proceeded at a furious pace, giving rise to far greater quantities of bilirubin than ever were seen in normal newborns. The destruction went on and on until the babies became profoundly anemic. Instead of being at rest, the bone marrow was in a frenzy of activity, spewing out red cells as fast as possible. In a frantic attempt to keep pace with the destruction, the marrow released into the blood great quantities of immature red cells, like an army swelling its dwindling ranks with boys after exhausting its reserves of men. The presence in the blood of large numbers of immature red cells, called erythroblasts, gave rise to the name, erythroblastosis, by which this condition is differentiated from all other forms of jaundice.

Either there was something wrong with the babies, which caused them to destroy normal red cells so voraciously, or there was something wrong with the red cells, which made them especially vulnerable to destruction. While others concentrated on trying to find a cause in the babies, Drs. Allen and Diamond concentrated on the red cells. They recognized that a process similar to what occurred in erythroblastotic babies was seen in some patients who accidentally received transfusions of the wrong blood type. How could there be a connection, since the babies had never been given transfusions before the destructive process began?

They knew that the fundamentals of blood typing had been worked out by testing the red blood cells of hundreds of people against thousands of serum samples. Sometimes when red cells were mixed with serum they became sticky and clumped together, whereas when mixed with the serum of other people they remained dispersed. They knew that the clumping was caused by the interaction of antigens on the surface of the red cells with antibodies in some of the serum samples. People whose cells had the most common antigen were called Group A. Those with the less common antigen were called Group B; those with both, Group AB and those with neither, Group O. A volunteer can donate blood to a patient safely only if his cells remain dispersed when mixed with the patient's serum. If this rule is broken, a reaction resembling that seen in erythroblastosis can occur.

Drs. Allen and Diamond knew that the serum of normal people never contains antibodies against their own red cells. They reasoned that the mother was the only source from which an unborn baby could receive foreign antibodies. But as far as A and B antibodies were concerned, the mother's blood was usually compatible with that of the baby so that reactions caused by A and B antibodies could not explain erythroblastosis in most cases. Perhaps there could be other antibodies.

When the red cells of humans were tested against animal serum all sorts of incompatibilities were found, but when the serum of monkeys was used a clear relationship was noted. Some human red cells clumped together in the serum of Rhesus monkeys, whereas others remained dispersed. All Rhesus monkeys had blood compatible with that of all other Rhesus monkeys, so the difference must lie not in them but in the humans against whom their serum was tested. This difference cut across all of the A, B, AB, and O blood types. Red cells from some people with each of these types clumped together in Rhesus monkeys' serum, while cells from others did not. A new blood-typing factor, the Rhesus monkey, or Rh factor, had been discovered. By using testing sera from both humans and Rhesus monkeys, human red cells could now be classified as type A, Rh positive, type B, Rh negative, and so on.

Dr. Allen noted that nearly all erythroblastotic babies had Rh positive cells while their mothers had Rh negative cells. These mothers with Rh negative cells did not normally have anti-Rh antibodies, but if they were given an Rh positive blood transfusion they slowly developed them, whereas Rh positive mothers never did.

Antibodies in the mother's blood can pass easily into the baby's blood across the thin membrane separating the two circulations in the placenta, but red blood cells are much too large to cross the placental barrier. Why did some Rh negative mothers develop Rh antibodies even though they had not been given a transfusion of Rh positive cells? Dr. Allen suspected, and was able to prove, that leaks sometimes occur allowing red cells from the baby to cross over into the mother's circulation. A mother's first Rh positive baby might thus stimulate her to begin making anti-Rh antibodies, but the baby was always safely out of the womb before she had time to make a harmful amount of them. Once she began to make them, she continued to do so for many years, thus jeopardizing any subsequent Rh positive babies she might conceive. Apparently leaks of Rh positive cells occurred quite frequently, acting as booster shots to induce the mother to produce more and more antibodies so that the risk to her Rh positive babies increased as the number of pregnancies increased.

Rh negative mothers were fortunate if their husbands were also Rh negative because all their babies were Rh negative. Some Rh positive fathers were capable of passing only Rh positive genes to their children whose red cells were always Rh positive. Some fathers whose own red cells were Rh positive were capable of passing either an Rh positive or an Rh negative gene to their children, so that occasionally a mother might have an Rh positive baby followed by an Rh negative one, and vice versa. Regardless of how severely affected her Rh positive child might be, the next one, if Rh negative, could not be harmed by the antibodies she had produced, nor could his red cells induce her to produce more antibodies.

That was the explanation for the devastating phenomenon of erythroblastosis. But what could be done about it? Dr. Allen concluded that the only way to stop the furious destruction of the baby's Rh positive cells was to remove them from the baby and replace them with a donor's Rh negative cells. By removing most of the baby's blood he could also drain out most of the antibody that the mother had passed on to him. The baby would gradually replace these donor cells with new Rh positive ones of his own, but by that time the remaining maternal antibody would wear out and be eliminated.

Ideally, one would first remove all of the baby's blood and then replace it with Rh negative blood, but this could not be done without killing the baby. The compromise was the exchange transfusion. About a third of an ounce of the baby's blood was removed and replaced by a like amount of donor blood. The process was repeated over and over until a whole pint of donor's blood was used. This is about twice as much as a full-term baby's body contains, and results in a thorough, but not quite complete, exchange of Rh positive cells for Rh negative ones.

Dr. Allen's exchange transfusions were becoming almost routine by the time I arrived at the Lying-In Hospital, and he had begun to allow us to do them ourselves. We typed every mother's blood when she went into labor. As soon as the baby's cord was cut some of the blood was taken from it for testing. It seemed odd to me at first that the blood from the cut end of a cord still dangling from the mother was the baby's blood and not hers, but of course it was.

If the baby's blood was Rh positive his serum was subjected to the Coombs' test, a simple test that showed the presence or absence of antibodies. Even if the baby's blood was Rh positive, a negative Coombs' test indicated that no damage had been done by prior exposure of the mother to Rh positive cells.

If the Coombs' test was positive, we tested the blood frequently for bilirubin, a test that fortunately requires only a few drops of blood and is easy to perform. If the bilirubin level began to rise rapidly, we performed an exchange transfusion at once. Time was of the essence because for some unknown reason the newborn baby's brain could not protect itself from low levels of bilirubin, levels that were not harmful to babies even a week or two old. Once the bilirubin had affected the brain, the damage was done, and although an exchange transfusion performed thereafter might save the baby's life, his brain would be severely damaged forever.

The hospital had a long list of eager volunteers with Rh negative blood. There were few uses of donor blood that had more appeal to those willing to give it than the saving of a newborn infant's life. The Rh negative mothers would have given anything to have us use their blood, and it was difficult to explain to them that even though they did have Rh negative blood it could not be used because it contained high levels of harmful antibody. Somehow, anesthesia, excitement, and the exhaustion of delivering a baby make a logical explanation of antibodies hard for a mother to comprehend.

Much has been done since 1954 to make exchange transfusions safer than they were then. We took all the precautions we could, but on looking back it seems remarkable to me that our primitive efforts produced no more damage than they did. Sometimes even repeating the procedure failed to save the baby, and I remember one who died after four exchange transfusions.

Nowadays exchange transfusions can be performed in virtually every hospital where babies are born, but in 1954 most erythroblastotic babies born in New England came to Boston for the procedure, often arriving pathetically late for us to do the baby much good. We never withheld exchange transfusion, even if brain damage was already obvious, and we sent home many babies so severely damaged that it might have been better to let them die untreated. This moral question and others like it plague all physicians who care for babies. The temptation to play God can be compelling, especially when the life in question has only just begun.

The new knowledge about the Rh factor was a boon to many families. Being forewarned by blood tests performed on the mother before delivery gave us the best chance to rescue the infant. This same knowledge was a tremendous source of anxiety for Rh negative mothers, and many who had little to worry about were consumed with fear concerning their unborn children. On Christmas Eve a mother came to the Lying-In Hospital in early labor. After the birth of her first Rh positive baby, who was perfectly normal, she had had five more Rh positive infants,

all of whom had died. Here she was again with Christmas only
hours away, convinced that she soon would lose a sixth. No
amount of reassurance could assuage her fear, and indeed her
prospects did look bleak. Unbeknownst to anyone, her husband
was one of those who could pass on either an Rh positive or an
Rh negative gene to his baby, and on Christmas morning she was
delivered of a beautiful, healthy Rh negative baby girl. She
thought it was a miracle, and so did I.

6

Who's Janice Greenough?

After our day's work was done, half of us stayed at the hospital all night while the rest went home to spend a few hours with our families before collapsing into bed. Spending thirty-six of every forty-eight hours together made the house staff a close-knit group, and was rewarding in many ways, but it deprived us of much contact with our children who were usually in bed before we got home. Fortunately, children who go to bed early get up early too, and we had precious times together before I went off to work. Jeff, who was going on five, was struggling mightily to stop wetting his bed. Early each morning when he had been successful his little blue eyes would peer around our door and he would announce triumphantly, "Hi Daddy, I did not wet my bed." One morning he appeared as usual and began, "Hi Daddy . . ." I waited in vain for him to continue. Finally, unable to stand the suspense, I ventured, "I did not wet my bed?" With utmost gravity he quietly confided, "I did not either."

Eleanor and Hardy Hendren who lived next door became great friends. Hardy was a surgical resident at Children's Hospital. He was a tremendous worker who loved surgery with all his heart and devoted even more hours to it than I did to medicine. He drove an old clunker with a hole in the muffler which roused the whole neighborhood when he drove off at dawn. If you lived next door to Hardy, you didn't need an alarm clock.

On the other side of the Hendrens lived Dr. and Mrs. Hermann. Our daughter, Amy, had a special bond with Dr. Hermann as they shared the same birthday. When Amy was two, Dr. Hermann was seventy-two. He was an erect and amiable giant who still practiced orthopedics every day. Until his retirement from academic affairs at sixty-five he had headed the famous Shortell fracture unit at Boston City Hospital. He bitterly resented having been forced to relinquish direction of this unit, and relished the fact that in the seven years since he had been "put out to pasture" three of his successors had died while he was still able to work. His career was remarkable in that while still a resident he had developed pernicious anemia. A young man with a growing family, he had become almost too weak to drag himself out of bed before his friend, Dr. Minot, discovered that injections of crude liver extract could correct the condition. Dr. Hermann was one of the earliest survivors, and as the refinement of vitamin B_{12} improved he was restored to vigorous and lasting good health. He and Mrs. Hermann had four sons and a daughter, all over six feet tall, and together they made a remarkable picture sharing his birthday cake with our tiny Amy. One of his sons was a professional wrestler who regaled the children with tales of victory over such heavyweight superstars as "Haystack" Calhoun.

Dr. and Mrs. Hermann had lived in their house for many years and had maintained it beautifully while the three around it had gradually suffered from lack of paint and overgrown bushes. The Hendrens had started a neighborhood rebirth, and a few weeks before we bought our house King and Ann Browne had begun fixing up the fourth. Dr. and Mrs. Hermann were delighted to have us all as neighbors and generally succeeded in making us forget that nearly a half century separated them from us.

King was a young lawyer who doubtless worked hard, but the fact that he was at home every night and on weekends was not lost on our children. One Sunday, as Patty drove them past the Browne's house on the way to share a hasty lunch with me at the hospital, Jeff remarked that it was too bad the Browne children only had a lawyer so they couldn't go to the hospital for lunch. Patty thought it was a cute remark, but I doubt if she recognized the volumes it spoke of the grace with which she handled being both mother and father so much of the time.

Once the outside of the house had been tidied up we went to work on the kitchen. The extra time I needed for this remodeling project was provided by a rotation at the hospital known as "night float." Unlike most other chiefs of his day, Dr. Janeway believed that house officers worked more efficiently and learned more if they got a reasonable amount of sleep. He assigned one of us at a time to a night rotation during which we "floated" from ward to ward attending to as many medical details as we could while the others slept. We came on duty at 11 P.M. just in time for the peanut-butter-and-jelly session where we were filled in on the day's activities, and we went home about nine in the morning after the first rounds of the day were over. In the dark hours we took first call for all medical problems in the emergency room and on the wards. We were not responsible for surgical patients, but often by restarting an intravenous infusion or ordering a medication for a child in pain we could spare a surgical or orthopedic colleague from being awakened. No one had more friends than an agreeable "night float."

The assignment had other advantages, including extra time to read and an unparalleled opportunity to watch emergency surgery. Hardy always let me know when surgery was about to start, and usually I could watch the important part of the operation before being summoned to another part of the hospital. With each operation I watched, the notion grew in my restless head that I should become a surgeon.

After my tour as "night float" I was scheduled to go to Salem for a rotation at the North Shore Babies' Hospital. While the experience would doubtless have been good for me, I dreaded the isolation from my family and eagerly accepted an extra tour as "night float" instead. By the time this second tour was over, the kitchen was finished, the dining room papered and painted, and a tiny room on the second floor paneled and fitted out as a study. Just when I thought I would have time to study up there I'm not sure, but the effort was not entirely wasted because Patty used it as a sewing room until Peter was born and took it over for his bedroom.

On my last night as "night float" I took my successor around
to show him the ropes and advised him of the value of helping
out the surgeons and orthopedists when the opportunity arose.
Evidently my pontification on this point sank in because on his
very first night he learned that one of the orthopedic patients
needed to have his intravenous infusion restarted. Whipping out
his scissors in the dimly lighted ward, he proceeded to remove
the adhesive tape holding the plugged needle in place and in the
process accidentally amputated the tip of the child's finger. The
disaster was compounded by the fact that the child was a
hemophiliac who needed the infusion so that he could receive
the clotting substance his body lacked. Only a few milimeters of
skin had been removed and the damage was promptly repaired
without repercussions of any sort, but the resident was so de-
moralized that he concluded he was unworthy to be a doctor
and insisted on quitting at once. Dr. Janeway canceled all appointments and sat with him for nearly twenty-four hours, patiently trying to convince him that despite this accident, he did
have a future in medicine after all. He finally relented and came
back to work, his medical career saved by a remarkable display
of compassion and sympathy. Dr. Janeway is a very special hero.

The first rule in vaudeville is never to follow a banjo act.
Campbell MacMillan was my banjo act. He preceded me on
every rotation, and every time he moved on people were sorry to
see him go. Not only was he a cheerful and very capable resident, but he had beautiful handwriting. These admirable qualities
especially endeared him to Dr. Alex Nadas, upon whose cardiology ward Campbell had done a particularly outstanding job.
Dr. Nadas was a somewhat walrus-shaped Hungarian who after
several years in a general pediatric practice had come to Children's Hospital to teach himself pediatric cardiology. So effectively had he availed himself of this opportunity that he was
widely held to be the foremost pediatric cardiologist in the
world.

There was a tremendous amount of work in children's cardiology. Rheumatic fever was still very common, and hundreds
of children with damaged hearts came to Dr. Nadas for medical
help. In addition, rapid strides were being made in heart surgery,
making accurate diagnosis of congenital heart defects suddenly

much more important than it had been in the past. The influx of cardiac patients was such that a whole floor was given over to them, with the surgical patients at one end and Dr. Nadas' medical patients at the other. The usual pattern was for children who needed heart operations to be admitted to the medical end where electrocardiograms, x-ray studies, and fluoroscopy were performed. After these diagnostic measures were finished the children were transferred to the surgical end. The lines of responsibility were very strictly drawn. Surgical patients were the surgeons' responsibility, medical patients were ours. Except in dire emergencies we never tended to the needs of surgical patients, and the surgeons never interfered with ours. This policy undoubtedly benefited the patients, and was perfectly acceptable to us as we had more than enough to do keeping up with the load of medical work.

Many of our patients were receiving daily doses of digitalis. Some children were much more sensitive than others to small doses of the drug, and disasters could occur if the early warning signs of digitalis overloading were overlooked. Dr. Nadas had developed charts listing these subtle signs and had one posted at the door of every child receiving digitalis. There was a column for each day of the week, and each day the resident filled in every little square in the proper column. Campbell's charts were works of art, and it was painfully obvious where his penmanship left off and mine began. On door after door hung chart after chart mutely proclaiming that Campbell MacMillan had been replaced by a lesser man.

Dr. Nadas never said anything to me about these wretched charts, but one afternoon word of his displeasure filtered down to me. I went home that night resolved to correct the deficiency the very next morning. An hour earlier than usual I arrived on the ward and carefully examined each of the eighteen children. Not waiting for a technician to appear, I took the electrocardiograph from bed to bed, obtaining fresh electrocardiograms from all of them. I took the charts down from the doors and made new ones, entering the fresh data I had obtained in the Friday column and painstakingly copying all of the data from Sunday through Thursday. At ten o'clock when Dr. Nadas stepped off the elevator to be taken on rounds he encountered the smug-

gest young resident in the history of medical training, convinced
beyond a shadow of a doubt that I could answer any question he
could possibly come up with.

"Good morning, Tom," said Dr. Nadas. "How's Janice Greenough?" I couldn't believe it. For five hours I had gone over
every child on the medical end of the floor. I knew them all by
heart, their histories, their heart murmurs, their electrocardiograms, how much digitalis they were taking, and everything
on every one of those miserable digitalis charts. There *was* no
Janice Greenough. I *couldn't* have missed her! Or could I?
Meekly I heard myself say, "Who's Janice Greenough?"

It turned out that Janice was the daughter of the hospital's
medical librarian, a dear friend of Dr. Nadas. She had been on
the medical end during Campbell's reign and had been transferred to the surgeons, operated upon, and discharged before I
had ever come to the floor. During the night, while I had been at
home, the surgeons had readmitted her with a fever of undetermined origin.

Dr. Nadas walked slowly over to me and put a heavy hand on
my shoulder. "Tom," he said, "aren't you interested?" A sledge-
hammer to the liver could not have hurt me more.

As soon as I could I withdrew to the washroom where I gazed
long and hard at my dejected self in the mirror. Why had he
hurt me so? Janice Greenough was not my responsibility. She
never had been. There was no reason in the world why I should
be expected to know she was back in the hospital. I should have
been able to tell him so with a totally unruffled conscience. But I
couldn't. Not because I didn't know who Janice Greenough was.
Not because he hadn't asked me any of the thousand questions I
was prepared to answer. Because he had hit the nail right on the
head. I *wasn't* interested in medicine. I wanted to be a surgeon.

7

A New Beginning

Once the decision to switch to surgery had been made, it was remarkably easy to carry out. I simply phoned for an appointment, drove over to Boston City Hospital for an interview, and was hired on the spot. Though I had never seen it before, there was something very familiar about Boston City Hospital. It looked, sounded, and smelled just like Bellevue. If anything, it was a little more drab and run down, with the hand of the politician a little more plainly visible. Most of the patients lay in long rows on open wards, though there were a few double rooms for the noisy, the politically favored, and the moribund. The wards were clean enough and reasonably bright on sunny days, but the various buildings were connected by feebly lit tunnels with crumbling walls and jagged cracks in the floors into which cockroaches scuttled furtively when anyone approached. One of these tunnels dipped down as it went under a street and at the bottom of the dip a series of planks made it possible to traverse a stagnant pool of water. The idea of keeping the water out by patching up the old concrete apparently never occurred to anyone with the authority to have it done.

The surgical patients were equally divided among three services. Dr. J. Englebert Dunphy ran the Harvard service. I felt he was using the position as a stepping stone, and would leave as soon as he was offered a more attractive post elsewhere. He soon did. Dr. J. J. Byrne headed the Boston University service. Completely at home in this niche, Dr. Byrne ran his service in an even-handed, low-key manner for the whole of his professional life. The morale of his house officers was serene and unruffled, and he had plenty of applicants for all of his training positions. Dr. Charles Gardner Child III had just arrived from Cornell, where I had known him slightly, to take the reins of the Tufts service. It was to Dr. Child that I poured out my longing to become a surgeon, and although I wasn't sure I told a very convincing tale, Dr. Child believed me. He convinced me that surgical training was so different from the pediatric training I had experienced that I should begin all over again at the very beginning—as an intern. If I were willing to do that, he could virtually guarantee that I would survive the pyramid and would eventually become his chief resident.

The pyramid was one of the major differences between pediatric and surgical training. In pediatrics nearly all the interns were kept on for two years of residency training and then became eligible to practice as qualified specialists. The surgical programs were five to seven years long, and only one of the eight who began as interns could be kept on for the final year as chief resident. Board certification in general surgery, a prerequisite to becoming a pediatric surgeon, could not be achieved without a chief residency. A number dropped out voluntarily along the way to go into specialties such as neurosurgery or orthopedics, but often the pyramid forced a cruel choice upon the department chairman who had to select one chief resident from among as many as four or five qualified people who had worked long and hard for him on the way up. Any hint that one would not be eliminated from the pyramid was rarely given, and I felt incredibly fortunate to receive this assurance from Dr. Child before I ever started to work for him.

Back at Children's the reserved and formidable Dr. Gross, from whom I hoped to receive advanced training in children's surgery later on, also accepted my yearning to switch to surgery as sincere. While agreeing that I was fortunate to have secured a place with Dr. Child, he carefully avoided making any commitment to me on his own part and left me with the distinct impression that while I had easily won the first half of the battle, the second half would be a different story.

Dr. Janeway accepted my decision to abandon his program gracefully enough. I never felt he knew me very well, but he chose to comment favorably on my handling of the tiny diabetic baby and to keep to himself any rumblings he might have heard from Dr. Nadas. We parted on good terms, no doubt in part because he had many applicants from whom to choose my replacement.

At home, the children were too young to grasp the implications of this change of plans, but Patty certainly did. Instead of one, or at most, two more years of struggling to stretch my meager salary and spending every other night alone, she could now look forward to at least five bleak years with no assurance that thereafter I would be successful in securing the training in pediatric surgery that was the whole point of the effort. The fact that Eleanor Hendren was cheerfully facing the same prospect next door was enormously helpful, but still it must have been very disheartening. Patty never showed her dismay, and never complained when I fell asleep almost before supper was over. My biggest regret is that I never found words to thank her then, and do not know how to do it even now.

My new internship began, as they all do, on July first, for the simple reason that medical schools turn their graduates loose in June. Was it really possible that only two short years ago I had looked as fresh and green and eager as the seven other interns did? Of course, they were all young enough to have escaped the military service that had interrupted my schooling for three years, so they were really five years younger than I. They never seemed to need to sleep.

The making of a surgeon differs sharply from that of a pediatrician. Pediatric training programs achieve a sense of progression and graded responsibility largely through giving the more junior people the less complicated assignments. Thus, I had progressed from malnutrition and diarrhea to leukemia and heart disease, always with patients of my own, and always considering my senior residents more as advisors than as bosses. The seniors were distinguished from the juniors mainly by the amount of administrative detail assigned to them. The chief resident drifted about the hospital, seeing the most interesting patients, making a helpful suggestion now and then, and scheduling teaching con-

ferences and the like. Dr. Holt's chief resident had even taken
time out to prepare an index for a pediatric textbook.

Surgical training much more closely resembles military service.
The interns are the privates; the assistant residents, the corporals;
and the chief resident, the sergeant major. The department chairman holds the chief resident accountable for every action of his
subordinates and for every detail of the care of all of the patients
on his service.

On any given day there were about fifty patients on our service, with peaks as high as seventy. A chief resident can only
bear this heavy burden of accountability by being very stingy
with the delegation of responsibility. Independent action, the
essence of medical training, is the antithesis of successful training in surgery. Anyone who has switched from a medical to a
surgical training program finds this constant suppression of ini-
tiative very hard to take.

Before Dr. Child's coming the service had been very loosely
run, and he regarded as his first priority the tightening up of dis-
cipline. Dr. Child would have made a superb general. He was
keenly interested in the progress of each one of us, but un-
failingly kept his distance from us in order not to undermine the
authority he had vested in his chief resident. We interns were
the only members of his house staff whom he himself had appointed, and a number of the senior residents knew full well that
they might not have been appointed at all had Dr. Child had any
say in the matter. Too many of them were motivated primarily
by fear of Dr. Child.

Our chief resident, Steve Meagher, was the best chief surgical
resident in the hospital. He had climbed to the top rung of the
ladder in the relaxed pre-Child era, and chafed constantly under
the tight rein with which Dr. Child kept him in check. Three afternoons a week Steve and his whole team took Dr. Child on
ward rounds. These were wonderful learning experiences for
those of us who didn't let fear of Dr. Child get the upper hand.
Our job was to present as succinctly as possible all there was to
know about each patient's problem and the results of all his lab
tests and x-rays. Steve would then outline his plan for treatment.
Dr. Child was a stickler for good English and could so squash an
intern's ego for a poor choice of words that he would be inca-

pable of learning anything for the rest of the day. I soon found out that my two years of practice in presenting cases gave me a great advantage, and after I found out what his pet grammatical peeves were, felt reasonably comfortable with Dr. Child.

These rounds were the bane of Steve's existence. He would worry all afternoon that one of us would let him down by forgetting some small detail, and he took Dr. Child's criticism of any of us as a personal wound. Time after time Steve would seek Dr. Child's approval to perform a major operation only to have his plan vetoed because the preoperative preparations had not met Dr. Child's exacting standards. Early in the year Steve lost about twenty pounds that he could ill afford to lose. We interns secretly suspected him of harboring an ulcer, but we never were able to catch him taking antacid tablets.

When Steve had finally surmounted all the obstacles Dr. Child had strewn in his path and arrived triumphantly in the operating room with a patient who was fully evaluated and carefully prepared, he was at last in his element. Dr. Child was a superb technician, but there was little he could show Steve about how to operate, and they both knew it. With Dr. Child as his first assistant Steve did operation after operation smoothly and skillfully. Eventually it dawned on Steve that Dr. Child poured so much energy into harassing him on the wards because he knew he had the makings of a very, very good surgeon. When Steve finally figured this out, it suddenly became fun to work for him.

Long before this momentous turning point Steve took me through my first operation. This was the moment I had been waiting for. I wanted it to be perfect, an operation the nurses would talk about, spreading the word that at last someone really good had been given a chance to show what he could do. I suppose I should have known it wouldn't turn out that way.

The patient was an ideal candidate for a neophyte's first effort, a lean and previously healthy teenager with early appendicitis. While Steve was busy elsewhere I had plenty of time to get him ready, and he arrived in the operating room with just the right amount of preoperative medication and an intravenous infusion taped in place with all the precision I could muster. Campbell MacMillan would have been proud of the chart I had prepared describing the history of his brief illness. The anesthetist scanned it approvingly and under his gentle ministration my first patient drifted effortlessly off to sleep.

I shaved his abdomen, meticulously swabbed it with iodine, and deftly applied the surgical drapes. Steve scrubbed his hands and arms for what seemed an eternity before taking up his place opposite me. The hour I had so long awaited was finally here. I was a surgeon at last.

Just at that moment, as so often happens when you least want it to, a couple of staff surgeons and a number of senior residents decided that they had nothing pressing to do and filed into the operating room to watch. I had participated in several appendectomies and thought I knew the procedure cold, but when the nurse thrust the knife into my hand my mind suddenly went blank and I couldn't for the life of me remember where to place the incision. Except for the rhythmic sounds of the patient's breathing and the steady drip of the intravenous the room was silent as a tomb. A hand came from behind me to wipe the sweat from my brow, and almost immediately it came back again. This wasn't the way it was supposed to be at all.

At last, convinced that no helpful hint was forthcoming from Steve, I made a tentative start, and step by painful step groped my way in an hour and a half through a procedure that should have taken no more than twenty minutes. When I finally sutured the edges of the incision together I thought it was the messiest job I had ever seen. The observers turned on their heels and departed without a word. Steve heaved a sigh of relief and followed them out the door. The scrub nurse who had patiently endured this dismal performance gathered up the instruments and started to put them away. As she handed me a bandage to cover my wrinkled incision she gravely lowered one eyelid and slowly raised it again. With no other acknowledgment, my first operation slipped into the oblivion it richly deserved.

All of the elective operations, those of a non-urgent nature which could be scheduled ahead, took place during the day Monday through Friday. Steve had expected to supervise or perform most of these without interference, as his predecessors had done. Dr. Child soon put a stop to this, insisting that he or one of his staff surgeons be present in the operating room during every elective operation. All the staff surgeons had private practices and cared for most of their patients in other hospitals. Few private patients were willing to put up with the primitive accommodations at the City Hospital, and therefore most of the time these staff surgeons spent there netted them no remuneration. I suppose each of them had his own reasons for devoting so much time to us, but their sacrifices constantly amazed me. One reason some of them did it was that the City Hospital offered an unparalleled opportunity to become expert at one type of surgery or another, and thus their private practices benefited indirectly. Dr. J. Edward Flynn spent hours and hours helping us to do all sorts of operations on the hand. He was a big burly man who was incredibly rough with delicate tissues, his roughness matched only by the speed with which he worked. Other more meticulous surgeons took three times as long to do comparable procedures, but Dr. Flynn's results were constantly better because he knew the anatomy of the hand, exactly where to find each little nerve and tendon, better than anyone else. Watching him work, I was convinced that the skin of the hand was to him as transparent as a glove of flexible glass. He was also intensely practical and took pains to find out all he could about what the patient expected to do with his hand once it had been repaired. Part of Dr. Flynn's genius was his ability to match his operations precisely to his patients' needs. As a result, he never sought perfection at the expense of realism, as I saw many other surgeons do. He would put a pianist through a long series of little operations stretched out over many months while for a laborer with the same condition, one long rough procedure would suffice. The laborer would be back at his unskilled work in a matter of days. Dr. Flynn loved life and had many keen perceptions about it. He also loved horses, and he liked me because I did too. I never got to ride one of his horses, but I'm sure they all had very hard mouths.

Donald Nabseth was a young surgeon interested in vascular surgery, which in those days was a far cry from the refined techniques of today. He dreamed of the day when coronary bypass operations would become feasible so that people with blockages in the arteries of their hearts could be restored to health. Before this goal could be reached surgeons would first have to learn how to bypass blockages in the vessels of the legs, and at Boston City Hospital Dr. Nabseth worked diligently to perfect this skill.

He was the opposite of Dr. Flynn, hesitant, patient, and endlessly careful. He was crisp and cool on the hottest summer day, and he had a hearty laugh which belied the total absence of a sense of humor. He had received all of his surgical training at Boston City Hospital and would go through his whole life repaying, through countless hours of devotion to helping the residents who came after him, a debt he perceived as impossible ever to repay in full.

The staff surgeon we most admired was Dr. John Crandon. Though he too had received some of his training at Boston City Hospital, he had long ago repaid any debt he might have felt he owed. He was a completely educated surgeon whose practice encompassed every type of general surgery. He had no special clinical hobbies, as Dr. Flynn and Dr. Nabseth had, and his practice was so huge and his reputation so secure that for the life of us we couldn't see what he had to gain by spending time with us. He did have a few private patients at the City Hospital, mostly priests, nuns, or nurses. We never resented the time we spent helping him care for his patients, feeling that he came closest of all our teachers to caring for his patients as we would want members of our own families to be cared for.

One of Steve's administrative tasks was to schedule operations at times when one of these staff surgeons could be present. This sometimes resulted in days or even weeks of delay for patients who otherwise were completely ready to be operated upon. One of my hardest tasks at Boston City was to tell patients that their operation had been canceled because no staff surgeon was available to supervise it.

At night and on weekends we endured another hardship. There were not enough scrub nurses to help us. Whenever there was none to be had, the job fell to the intern. Though we hated playing the role of scrub nurse, handing instruments up the line and threading needles instead of being able to watch or help with the operation, we learned a great deal of surgery acting as scrub nurses. I am convinced that no surgeon can fully appreciate a good scrub nurse unless he has served in that capacity himself. Nowadays interns practically never get the opportunity to do so.

Unlike the elective procedures, which Dr. Child insisted be chaperoned by a staff surgeon, the only requirement for emergency cases was that a staff surgeon be informed as to what the resident perceived the problem to be and what he proposed to do about it. Steve had made himself thoroughly familiar with the whims and life-styles of the various staff surgeons, and he constantly scanned the list for one who could be reached at home or at his club, but could be counted on not to show up in person. Whenever the emergency operation was minor enough to delegate to a junior resident, Steve had the option to decide whether or not to be present in the operating room. He had a keen sense of what his juniors were capable of and rarely got surprised, but Guy Leadbetter and I provided him with a very unpleasant exception.

Guy had just finished his internship when I arrived on the service. He was a very bright and aggressive junior resident with a keen interest in urology. He came by this interest naturally enough, as his uncle was Chief of Urology at Massachusetts General Hospital. He had never done any of the really big general surgical operations, but this never daunted him.

Late one Saturday afternoon I admitted a frail old man with a huge abscess on the back of his neck. We told Steve about it, and he in turn told a staff surgeon who was about to play a tennis match and would cause us no trouble. With Steve's blessing Guy and I took the old gentleman to the operating room to drain the abscess.

The anesthetist, who was as green as we were, pasted a stethoscope on the old man's chest, wrapped a blood-pressure cuff around his arm, and slipped him a load of pentothal. He was asleep in an instant and we rolled him onto his side to gain better access to the back of his neck. Wishing to be as helpful as possible, the anesthetist pushed the old man's head forward so that his chin rested on his chest, unwittingly shutting off his ability to breathe.

Oblivious to the impending disaster, I painted the skin with iodine and covered the old man's head with sterile drapes. Just as Guy was donning his gloves the anesthetist let out a mournful groan and announced that the patient's heart had stopped beating. Acting as if this happened several times in an average day, Guy calmly ripped off the towels covering the old man's face. It was a ghastly blue. He was as dead as a doornail.

Pushing me and the anesthetist aside, Guy rolled the patient onto his back and plunged the knife meant for the abscess into his chest. In seconds he had made a gash ten inches long. The edges of this huge incision didn't bleed at all. Forcing the two biggest retractors we had into the wound, Guy yelled at me to pull. As the ribs separated we saw the heart, full, motionless, and deep, deep blue. While the anesthetist rhythmically inflated the old man's lungs Guy alternately squeezed and released the heart. It took only a few puffs of oxygen and a few of Guy's vigorous squeezes to get it going again, and I watched in amazement as it contracted, first slowly and feebly, then faster and more forcefully. The dark blue color lightened to a normal red, and Guy began to suture up the wound. I glanced at the clock. The whole drama had consumed less than three minutes.

When the wound was partially closed Guy inserted a chest tube, a red rubber hose about as big as his little finger. The purpose of this big tube, whose tip would lie inside the chest for several days, was to remove the air surrounding the lung so that it would remain fully expanded.

"Now," said Guy, "we need some suction bottles." These are a series of three large glass bottles attached to each other by small rubber hoses. From the first, a long rubber hose connects to the tube in the patient's chest, and from the last a short tube leads to a small electric pump. The chest tube, the bottles, and the pump are standard equipment.

The nurse calmly informed us that there were none. Every set was in use by a patient who could not give it up. When you have a problem the nurse can't handle you go to the supervisor. We paged the supervisor. We paged again. And again. Being four o'clock on Saturday afternoon we should have looked in the little kitchen off the surgical ward where the supervisor was having her customary cup of tea with the priest. Instead, we badgered the telephone operator who kept bleating ineffectually into the loudspeaker until the ritual was over and the teacups washed and put away. When the supervisor finally appeared, smoothing her feathers like a mother hen who had been caught in a rainstorm, she gave us the same answer. There simply weren't any chest tube bottles to be had.

At the City Hospital, when all else failed, you went to the

Exec. The Exec. was the court of last appeal. He was a doctor appointed by the politicians to make things run smoothly. He settled disputes between residents of different services and saw to it that the politically favored got a bed when beds were scarce. No doctor with an ounce of intelligence would take the job. Dr. Magner did. Nobody knew why.

We stormed into his office to find him engrossed in the evening newspaper. Eventually he became aware of our presence and asked us, rather defensively I thought, what he could do for us. Guy calmly recited our tale, how we had taken a patient to the O.R. for an emergency operation, how his heart had stopped, how we had opened his chest, massaged his heart and got it going again, and how we needed chest tube bottles to keep his lungs expanded, and how we had exhausted all available resources before disturbing Dr. Magner. Guy modestly failed to mention the fact that had it not been for his quick thinking and bold action there would be no problem for Dr. Magner about finding chest tube bottles, but some very sticky questions for him to answer to the coroner instead. Dr. Magner listened silently to Guy's recital, pursed his lips, and after a long pause murmured, "But Doctor, it's five o'clock. You should have planned on this!"

8

Rotations

We interns spent about half the year on the "home team," helping Steve care for his patients, and the other half on rotations. On my first rotation I was assigned to the emergency room. I loved this rotation because, in addition to the many adults, I had a chance to care for a few children. I hadn't realized how much I missed them.

There was a senior resident to handle the complicated cases, so my job did not involve high-level decisions. My function was to handle minor problems such as cuts and bruises. I had a tiny operating room in which to sew up people, and was assisted by a self-taught technician who worked as a hairdresser at night and was saving up money from his two jobs to open his own beauty shop. John had a wonderful way with patients and could tape the edges of many jagged lacerations together with butterflies better than even a plastic surgeon could suture them. He made the butterflies himself by cutting and folding little pieces of adhesive tape so that the ends were still sticky while the middle portion was not.

One day a policeman brought in a little boy with a small cut on his lip. I sat on a stool at the head of the stretcher holding the boy's head and murmuring soothing messages in his ear while John prepared to work his magic with the butterfly. Like most policemen, this one was interested in what went on in an emergency room, and it never occurred to me to ask him to leave. He took up a position behind me and watched as John put in a little Novocain and washed out the cut. The little boy's mother arrived and watched from the foot of the table. Everything seemed to be going smoothly until John decided to improve on perfection by trimming the butterfly he had stuck in place. He whipped out his scissors, pulled up on the tape, and cut a gash in the little boy's lip about three times as big as the cut he had come in with. The whole lip was numb with Novocain, and the boy didn't move or say a word. The mother, whose view was blocked by John's shoulder, was blissfully unaware of the accident. Since she had never gotten a clear view of the cut in the first place, I was sure we were home free. All John would have to do was to stick on another butterfly and nobody would be the wiser. The policeman, who had seen the whole thing, worked for the same City of Boston we did, and would never betray us, I was sure. It wasn't until he blurted out, "Oh, Jesus, you cut him!" that I realized the worst. The policeman was the little boy's father.

A football player, all of five years old, came in with a nasty gash he had sustained on the field of strife. As I was cleaning his wound, I asked him casually what position he played. "Tangle," he replied. Little boys are keenly aware of their roles in life.

One afternoon a brave little lad arrived clutching a very dead snake with the flattest head I had ever seen. We phoned the museum and were told that the snake was not poisonous. The boy announced that he hadn't thought it was, and had only come to the hospital because his mother made him. The snake had bitten him on the hand, he said, and that had made him mad, so he had picked up a rock and bashed its head in. John found an old jar of formalin in which to preserve it, and the reluctant patient departed with a Band-Aid on his finger, proudly bearing his trophy with which to regale his classmates and scare his teacher. I hope she was properly horrified.

Among the pesky little problems we had to deal with were toothaches. There was a dentist whom we could call if all else failed, but we were supposed to do everything we could before disturbing him. Many of the patients had terribly neglected teeth with huge cavities. We could often relieve their pain temporarily by dropping in a few drops of "Boston City Hospital Toothache

Remedy." This was mainly oil of clove which had a strong me-
dicinal smell and dulled the pain for a few minutes. We soon
learned that it was most effective if put in the cavity just before
a streetcar was due to pass by the hospital. The patient would
express profound gratitude that his pain was gone and would be
well on his way home before it returned.

We worked as fast as we could so as not to get too far behind,
because the sooner we started to take care of a patient's problem
the less complaining we would hear. We failed to get to one little old lady soon enough, however, and while she was waiting
for someone to give her something for constipation, she fell off
her stretcher and broke her hip. Three months later I happened
to meet her hobbling down the corridor to the discharge office. I
tried to hide before she recognized me, but I was too late, and
she thanked me profusely for being so kind to her when she had
come to the hospital.

After I left the emergency room I spent two months giving
anesthesia. Dr. Dunphy had already taken the Harvard interns
off this valuable rotation, and in a few years most surgical programs would drop it. It was a great loss. The argument was that
anesthetists didn't learn to operate, so why should surgeons learn
to give anesthesia? The fact is that anesthetists know a lot more
about surgical technique than most surgeons do about anesthesia.
It is very difficult to learn much about anesthesia while performing operations. On the other hand, anesthetists watch surgical
procedures day after day, and in teaching hospitals hear over and
over the reasons for doing things in a certain way. Often an anesthetist, alert to a problem I was facing, has helpfully suggested
that he had seen another surgeon handle a similar situation in a
way that hadn't occurred to me. They only tell you if they
think you'll listen.

Ether was the usual anesthetic agent. Nowadays nobody has to
endure the slow, suffocating torture of being put to sleep with
ether, but in the hands of the inexperienced no modern anesthetic is as safe as ether was. The very slowness with which it
acted was its chief virtue. It took forever to get a patient anesthetized deeply enough for the surgeon to be able to begin to
work, but at least we had plenty of time to recognize that we
were pushing it too far before it was too late.

To speed the induction of sleep we often started with Vinethene. Like ether, Vinethene was a vile smelling liquid that vapor-
ized when poured over an ether mask. Once he got a whiff of
Vinethene the patient usually held his breath as long as he could.
Finally, with suffocation the only alternative, he would suck in a
huge breath and go into a paroxysm of coughing which made
further breath-holding impossible. Every available hand was
required to hold the struggling victim on the table until he
finally surrendered to the noxious vapor and dropped off to
sleep. This phase of excitement was followed by one charac-
terized by deep, rapid respirations, during which we made the
switchover to ether. Every anesthetist juggling a Vinethene bottle, a can of ether, and an ether mask at the same time has wished
he had three hands. If the Vinethene were stopped before the patient became saturated with ether, he would promptly wake up
and start struggling again. If we kept pouring on the Vinethene
too long his heart would become wildly irregular, and sometimes
stop altogether. In the hands of a skilled anesthetist it looked easy
enough, but it wasn't.

As soon as we became reasonably proficient with Vinethene
and ether we were taught to give spinals. A needle was introduced into the spinal canal where the roots of the nerves supplying the lower half of the body are bathed in spinal fluid. We
could tell that the needle was in proper position when a few
drops of crystal clear spinal fluid dripped from it. Pontocaine
was injected, the needle quickly withdrawn, and the patient
helped to sit up. The Pontocaine, being heavier than spinal fluid,
sank to the bottom of the spinal canal. In about five minutes the
anesthetic was "set," and the patient could be put flat without
fear that the agent would travel upward to paralyze the nerves
which controlled his breathing. As soon as he was made comfortable and became convinced that he really could not feel what
the surgeon was doing, he usually dropped off to sleep. Our job,
once the operation began, was simply to monitor the blood pressure. The staff anesthetists could hardly wait for us to learn to
do spinals, which were usually very simple and invariably bor-
ing.

Perhaps the ideal operation for a spinal anesthetic was hip
nailing. There were lots of them—two or three hip nailings a

day were not uncommon. The patients were always elderly, often with medical problems that made it risky to use ether. They usually believed that they had fallen and broken their hips, but in reality the bone had given way and caused the fall. The operation was a boon to these fragile old people because it allowed them to get out of bed and move about, greatly reducing their chances of getting bed sores or pneumonia.

The usual plan was to schedule one staff anesthetist to supervise two adjacent operating rooms. In one, a complicated operation under ether would occupy most of his attention, while in the other the intern gave custodial care to a patient with a spinal. Such were the circumstances when I gave my first solo performance with spinal anesthesia.

My patient was a little old lady who must have existed for years on tea and toast. Soaking wet she weighed no more than ninety pounds. I hit the target on the first try; clear spinal fluid dripped from the hub of the needle. I drew four miligrams of Pontocaine into a small syringe. The staff anesthetist was searching frantically in the wall cabinet for some piece of equipment with which to stave off disaster next door. I got his attention long enough to secure his approval of the dose I had selected. He gave me a quizzical look, which I interpreted to mean that six would be better, and scurried out the door. Actually he was thinking that two would probably be plenty. I injected six, withdrew the needle and sat the old lady up. It was like lifting an empty egg box. After a suitable time I laid her down and pricked her leg with a pin. As I expected, she did not feel a thing. The surgeon painted her skin with iodine. I saw her lips form a silent prayer, and then she fell asleep.

The operation went smoothly. Why shouldn't it? You could practically see the break in the bone under her skin. I was sitting there, fat, dumb, and happy when Dr. Marcus silently appeared at my elbow. Like most chiefs of anesthesia, Dr. Marcus had developed an uncanny knack for showing up where trouble was about to happen. He gave my little lady a brutal pinch on the shoulder and said in a loud voice, "Cough, Mother!" "Cough?" she replied, almost inaudibly, "I can't even open my mouth!" Dr. Marcus slapped a mask over her face and set me to rhythmically squeezing a rubber bag filled with oxygen. "She'll need this for a while." It was a masterpiece of understatement. The operation ended six hours before my generous dose of Pontocaine had worn off so that she could breathe on her own. But for Dr. Marcus' timely arrival she would have had little need for a nail in her hip.

The final two months of my internship were spent on pathology. We had studied pathology early in medical school, and most of us had decided we never wanted anything to do with it again. Pathology is the study of abnormal anatomy. Like spinach, pathology is good for surgeons, though it takes a long time to get to like it. Distasteful as some aspects of pathology may be, it is impossible to imagine surgery having matured from the crude efforts of the ancient barbers to the modern science it has become without the aid of pathologists. In the operating room their rapid decisions as to whether a tumor is benign or malignant guide the surgeon in selecting the operation best calculated to help his patient. In the autopsy room the lesson the pathologist learns no longer helps the patient whose body gives up the secret, but it may benefit countless others who come after.

In two short months we could not be exposed adequately to pathology in both the operating room and the autopsy room. Since we would encounter pathologists daily in the operating room for the rest of our lives, our rotation consisted of two months of duty in the autopsy room.

Nobody enjoys witnessing his first autopsy, but actually doing his first one is even worse. I seriously doubted that I could go through with it. I had visions of my surgical career foundering right there in the autopsy room. A little lack of sympathy on the part of my instructor and it would have been all over. Fortunately, he knew just how to handle the situation, and before I knew it, I had begun. Anticipation was much worse than action, and once a start had been made I was able to continue.

In all, I did thirty-seven autopsies during that May and June. From them I learned anatomy as I had never understood it before. The spatial relationships of one body part to another are much more difficult to remember when viewed through the limited access of a surgical incision than through the much wider one an autopsy provides. A surgeon who has mastered anatomy can make his way quickly and surely to a target deep within the body because in his mind's eye he can see it through the intact skin. This only comes from opening the skin, fixing the structures beneath it firmly in mind, and continuing to see them vividly after the skin has been closed over them again. Hour after hour in the autopsy room we doggedly repeated this simple exercise, and the knowledge we acquired stuck with us for the rest of our lives.

9

The Telegram

With our intern rotations behind us, we returned to the "home team" as junior residents. We had climbed the first rung of the ladder. One of our group had gone off to another training program, and Dr. Child had gotten Chris Economopoulis to take his place. To nobody's surprise Chris announced that he was from Greece.

Chris had a sister who was studying to become a pediatrician, and the two of them were planning to return to their home city in Greece where she would head the department of pediatrics and he would be the pediatric surgeon. As Chris explained it, competition for these politically appointed positions was fierce, and the chance that one of them would be successful was very slim. The chances of a brother and sister team landing both of these plums were about one in a million, but if determination had anything to do with it these two would reduce the odds against them to fifty-fifty. None of us had ever met a harder worker than Chris Economopoulis.

Chris should have been a boon to us, but he wasn't. Nobody could help him. He insisted on doing everything himself. His constant refrain in defense of this compulsion was, "I have to learn." If we heard it once we heard it a thousand times a day. Boston City wasn't overly generous with supplies like adhesive tape, but it must have been profligate compared to the hospital Chris came from. On the fourth of July, three days after his arrival, Chris insisted on starting all the intravenous infusions on the ward. There were at least twenty of them, and I began the day thinking what a luxury it was going to be to have this diligent soul on our team. Chris eventually got them all going, but he was so parsimonious with the tape that none of them stayed in place very long, and by nightfall I had restarted every last one of them.

These middle years, between internship when everything was new and different and the final year when as chief resident we would do the big operations, were mainly years of learning by watching. Hopefully we would see mistakes along the way which we would not repeat when our turn came. One day a severely malnourished little old lady was brought in to our service. Her daughter had taken her to a local hospital because of vomiting, and a surgeon had operated on her to bypass a narrowing caused by a duodenal ulcer. After the operation she had never vomited again, but instead of gaining weight she had gone steadily downhill until she was little more than skin and bones. She could not get out of bed without help, and could walk only a few steps.

Dr. Child took one look at the short scar on her abdomen and at once suspected what the trouble was. We took her to the X-ray Department and gave her a swallow of barium. On the fluoroscope we watched it leave her stomach, pass through about eight inches of small intestine and promptly appear in her colon. The barium should have taken at least two hours to reach the colon. On the way it should have traversed three yards of small intestine, but as Dr. Child had predicted, the surgeon had bypassed nearly all of it. He had simply made too short an incision to allow himself to see what he was doing. The real horror was not that he had done the operation improperly, but that he hadn't recognized his mistake and corrected it. Before we could prepare her for the simple operation that would have set her on the road to recovery, she gave her daughter a wistful smile, turned her face to the wall, and died. From then on nobody had to tell me to make my incisions big enough so that I could see what I was doing.

Surgical training takes a long time, and there are very few shortcuts on the way to the all-important chief residency, but it was possible to substitute one year of pediatric surgery for twelve months of general surgery—if you could get it. There were only about a dozen training programs in pediatric surgery in the entire country, and the one at Boston Children's Hospital was by far the most sought after. A bachelor might go off for a year to Chicago or Seattle, but for me, with a wife, three children and a fourth on the way, it was Boston or nothing. The fact that I was an alumnus of sorts, having spent a year in pediatric medical training there, didn't give me any advantage at all with the surgeons.

I had tried repeatedly to get an opportunity to discuss my future with Dr. Gross. His secretary was always polite, always remembered that I had called before, but steadfastly refused, presumably on orders from on high, to give me an appointment. Three letters went unanswered.

Dr. Gellis, whose attention I had attracted early in my medical year at Children's, happened to overhear me bemoaning my lack of communication with Dr. Gross.

"He won't pay any attention to letters and phone calls," he said. "You have to do something unusual. Why don't you send him a telegram?" I had to admit it was an avenue I hadn't explored.

I spent several days mulling over possible messages and finally settled on the following: "ROBERT E. GROSS M.D. BOSTON CHILDREN'S HOSPITAL BOSTON MASS STOP HAVE CONTACTED YOUR OFFICE MANY TIMES FOR APPOINTMENT STOP NO REPLY STOP HOLT JANEWAY CHILD ALL PLEASED WITH MY WORK STOP MAY I COME STOP TOM MORSE"

The lady behind the desk at the Western Union office could not resist the temptation to remind me that Boston Children's Hospital was less than half a mile from where we stood. I assured her that it might as well be a million miles away when it came to reaching it by mail or telephone, and she wished me luck as I paid for my telegram. I remember that I gave her a dollar and she gave me some change. I have forgotten how much.

Whatever the cost, it did the trick. Two weeks later, at ten o'clock at night, Dr. Gross called me from his office to say that he had an opening for me if I would come at once. Someone who was supposed to be coming from Sweden had run into visa trouble. I agreed to come over and give him my answer in the morning.

I was sure Dr. Child would not let me go on such short notice. He needed every one of us, and had agreed to let me go at the end of the year only if he could find a replacement for me. To find someone who wanted one year of general surgical training in a program that had no room to keep him on thereafter was not easy. To find a substitute who could start at once in the middle of the year would be impossible. My big break had come, but it had come too soon.

Dr. Child was not overjoyed at the prospect of going through the rest of the year shorthanded, but he did not refuse to let me go. Instead of making the decision, he turned it back to me, advising me to try to determine from Dr. Gross whether or not I might get another chance if I turned this offer down. If I felt this would be my only chance, Dr. Child advised me to take it. Few other chiefs of surgery, at least in that era, would have been as generous.

My meeting with Dr. Gross lasted less than two minutes. It was like a quick appointment with the Sphinx. I knew he had no way of knowing whether or not another opportunity to take me on would come along, and I was reasonably sure he wouldn't say so if he did. On my way over from the City Hospital I had decided there was no way I could take the job. He accepted my decision without comment, and I left without having heard anything to indicate what he was thinking. But something in his eye told me I had done the right thing.

I had never seen Patty so dismayed as she was when I told her what I had done. Knowing how much it meant to me, she simply couldn't believe I could be so dumb as to turn this wonderful offer down. I certainly didn't have any right to expect another one. Despite the fact that she was making every bit as great a sacrifice as I was, it hadn't even occurred to me to discuss it with her before I had decided what I was going to do. My colleagues at Boston City were certain I had lost my mind. But Dr. Child was very grateful, and in due time a second offer from Dr. Gross did come. This time there was ample time to find a replacement for me and I accepted the offer eagerly, my future with Dr. Child secure.

10

Pediatric Surgery

I had been away from Boston Children's Hospital for less than two years, but my first reaction on returning was surprise that there were so few familiar faces. Most of the pediatric residents with whom I had worked were gone. A number of them, I remembered ruefully, were well into their first year of private practice.

During the peanut-butter-and-jelly sessions I had acquired a pretty accurate knowledge of what lay in store for me. It bore little resemblance to private practice. I was starting at the bottom for the third time. I would be known as a junior resident, but for the next eight months there would be nobody under me. Call me what you will, I was once again an intern.

For the first two months I would be known as the "pup." It would be my job to start intravenous infusions, draw blood samples for the lab, get x-rays in order for conferences, and do a host of similar joyless but necessary tasks. Only in dire emergencies would I be pressed into service in the operating room.

At the end of two months a new "pup" would appear, and I would move on to the private service. There was little risk that I would make many wrong decisions on the private service. The staff surgeons made all the decisions. During these first four months I would also cover the emergency room.

Next I would move to a two-month rotation on neurosurgery, more because the neurosurgeons needed a body than because I needed an education in neurosurgery, I thought. As will be seen, I later changed my mind. Thereafter I would be assigned to the cardiac service, where for the first time I would come into daily contact with Dr. Gross. During these eight months I would do practically no operating, but if I could organize my chores efficiently, I could do a fair amount of watching from the galleries and hopefully would learn how things were supposed to work. For the final four months I would return to the chief resident's service where now somebody else would be "pup."

The fact that each of us took these rotations in the same order was of great advantage to Dr. Gross, but this neat progression could only be achieved if a new resident joined the service every two months. Since the rest of the world worked on a different schedule, Dr. Gross found great difficulty in persuading chiefs of surgery around the country to release a man here and a man there when he could fit them in. It would be much simpler if he could get all six of his junior residents from the same hospital. Dr. Gross persuaded Dr. Francis Moore of the Peter Bent Brigham Hospital to work out a schedule allowing him to do just that, and thereafter for several years the door was closed to junior residents from all other hospitals. The arrangement went into effect four months after my "pupship" began.

The real significance of this agreement was the effect it could be expected to have on Dr. Gross' selection of senior residents. Two years of training at this level were necessary if one wanted to practice pediatric surgery. The chief resident was always chosen from among these senior residents, and it seemed only logical that the senior residents would tend to be selected from among the six junior residents who started each year as "pups." That was why I had wanted the appointment so desperately. I knew I was tremendously fortunate to get it, but since Dr. Gross' agreement with Dr. Moore had not yet been announced, I did not know how miraculously close I had come to being shut out altogether.

Pediatricians, especially those on medical college faculties, were clamoring for more trained pediatric surgeons. It was reliably predicted that within the next ten or fifteen years every medical school in the country would have at least one pediatric surgeon on its staff. Responsible positions in this challenging field were falling to Dr. Gross' trainees as fast as he could turn them out.

In addition to the leadership of Dr. Gross and the handful of pediatric surgeons at work in other centers, two factors for which they were not responsible were propelling pediatric surgery to an importance it had never known before. The first was the improved safety of all kinds of surgery. Widespread acceptance of blood transfusions and safer anesthesia were making it possible to perform with little risk operations that only a few years before would have been attended by a prohibitive mortality. The second was the dwindling importance of medical illness as a killer of children. Malnutrition, infant diarrhea, and contagious diseases no longer dotted family grave plots with tiny headstones. Antibiotics such as sulfonamides and penicillin made it possible to cure thousands of children who formerly would have died of pneumonia or other infections. As one pediatric threat after another fell before the advance of medical knowledge three major killers remained. Together they now claimed the lives of more than half of all children who died before reaching adulthood. They were injury, cancer, and congenital malformations, and they were all surgical problems.

As the field of pediatric surgery evolved, each of these major child-killers would in turn occupy center stage. Life-threatening injury, statistically the most significant of the three, is only now beginning to receive the attention it deserves. Cancer was still at a stage in which early recognition was far more important than any skill the surgeon might have. The work that Sidney Farber was pioneering in chemotherapy would soon greatly increase the role of the surgeon in dealing with cancer in children, but as with trauma, cancer's time for center stage had not yet come.

The pediatric surgeon was first and foremost an expert in correcting congenital malformations. Some of these, including most correctable heart deformities, were best repaired when the children were between two and ten years old. Others, like diaphragmatic hernias, were rapidly fatal if not corrected within minutes after birth. A very large group involved malformations of the intestine. Though these did not require quite the stampede to the operating room that diaphragmatic hernias did, they needed deft and expert operative correction within the first forty-eight hours of life because until they were repaired the infant could not begin to eat. Not only must the surgeon's operation permit the infant to live in comfort and maintain his body weight, which is all that is required of intestinal surgery in adults, but it must also provide for normal growth and development. It was mastery of the management of life-threatening congenital malformations in infants and children that distinguished the pediatric surgeon from all others. As the new "pup," I stood on the threshold of this exciting world.

The chief resident for whom I went to work was Lester Martin. Two years before, Lester had encouraged me to switch to surgery, and he welcomed me to his service with his huge friendly grin. He was a born leader, strong, practical, and very kind. In a few months he would finish his ninth year of surgical training. Lester ran his service with total autonomy. Dr. Gross had complete confidence in him, and made ward rounds with him only once a week.

Lester gave me a list of chores to do and told me to be sure to be ready at noon because this was Dr. Gross' day to be taken on rounds. Back at City Hospital I had never thought of Dr. Child as garrulous, but he was downright chatty compared to the reserved and taciturn Dr. Gross. We moved from crib to crib about as fast as we could walk, Lester summing up each child's problem in a word or two, Dr. Gross responding with a nod or a grunt. Lester knew what each of these nods and grunts meant and would explain them to us later.

There seemed to be three reasons why Dr. Gross was able to teach so much while saying so little. One was that he was perhaps the most consistent surgeon ever born. Having shown how to do something once, he expected it to be done precisely that way on every subsequent occasion. This remarkable consistency made it easy for residents to function as his disciples, each passing the wisdom of the master surgeon to the next resident down the line.

The second was his classic textbook, *The Surgery of Infancy and Childhood.* Published in 1953, the year I started at Bellevue, it presented in minute detail the surgical experience of the Boston Children's Hospital over a fifteen-year period during which more than thirty thousand infants and children had been operated upon. Many of its chapters described larger groups of similar cases than had ever before been reported in the world's literature. Dr. Gross had ensured consistency by writing every word of the final text himself, although many people had contributed by digging up statistics and putting rough drafts together. Now nearly thirty years old, it is still considered one of the finest texts ever published on any medical subject. Some parts of it are very out of date today, but it was only three years old when I began to read it, and at that time it reflected the most modern surgical care of infants and children. I read and reread it many times, and to this day know long passages of it by heart.

Perhaps most important was Dr. Gross' ability to get people to do their best for him. He never sought respect; it fell to him naturally. In all the time I worked for him I never saw him ruffled, never heard him raise his voice to anyone, never heard him ask anyone to work hard for him. It just never occurred to anyone not to. When we assisted him in the operating room he often performed an operation from start to finish without saying a word. But we sensed the passionate intensity with which he wanted everything he did to be perfect, and we worked our hearts out for him, because we wanted it to be perfect too.

Though many who had preceded me in the role of "pup" knew more general surgery than I did, they often had had little or no experience in caring for babies. I was completely at home in meeting many of the babies' basic needs, such as feeding formulas and intravenous infusions. Lester thought I was a pretty respectable "pup" and kept his eye open for a way to reward me. After about six weeks a suitable opportunity presented itself.

On a busy Friday afternoon a very sick child with a ruptured appendix arrived in the emergency room. To make room for him on the operating schedule, Lester bumped a little girl with an umbilical hernia, promising her mother to reschedule the operation for the following day. On Saturday morning, while Lester and I were going over my list of chores for the day, the operating room called to ask who was supposed to repair the little girl's hernia. Lester was mortified. He had forgotten all about her. He told the operating room not to page anyone, he would handle it himself.

"Tom," he said, "go down there and get it started. I'll grab a bite of breakfast and be right down to help you." At Boston City Hospital that would have translated, "Go as far as you can as fast as you can, because if you're nearly finished when I get there I may let you continue, but if you're just getting started I'll take over and do the operation myself."

In the operating room there were always visitors from other hospitals, and today was no exception. Pressed up against the wall so as to be as inconspicuous as possible was a little nurse from England. I later found out that she worked in the operating room of the Hospital for Sick Children in London, the foremost children's hospital in the British Empire. Ignoring her completely, I flew into my gown and gloves and began to sterilize the skin of the little girl's abdomen. As I completed this antiseptic maneuver and was starting to apply the sterile drapes a wee voice with a very British accent inquired, "Don't you want to dip it in the iodine?" So intent had I been on beginning my *tour de force* that I had been wiping the skin with a swab of dry cotton!

Many of the infants and children we looked after came from Boston or one of its suburbs, and their parents could visit them fairly regularly. However, many others came from far away, and for their parents we conducted a telephone hour at seven o'clock every evening. These sessions really kept us on our toes because we never knew which parent the operator would put on the line next. I lived in fear of accidentally giving bad news about one child to the parents of another, or unintentionally misleading the parents of a child who was doing poorly that all was well. So far as I know, I never got mixed up, but I never felt comfortable until the telephone hour was over. The experience was hard on the parents too. Many of them waited on the line for nearly an hour night after night to have a few words with a doctor they had never met. Putting myself in their places, I marveled at their bottomless faith in us.

Nowhere was the contrast with Boston City Hospital more striking than in the emergency room. The spacious surroundings, the sparkling cleanliness, and the abundance of nursing help made it a delight to work there—most of the time. I did have one uncomfortable moment there late one night. The waiting room was empty and the lights turned down low, when through the door burst a harried general practitioner carrying a limp and obviously critically ill baby. He thrust the baby into my arms, shouting that the father was following in another car and would be here any moment.

"He says he'll kill the doctor if the baby dies. Better you than me, son!" He bolted out the door.

The father did indeed appear less than a minute after this hasty departure. He had apparently cooled down considerably on the way to the hospital. The Al Capone I had been expecting was just a typical father after all, frightened and pathetically helpless in his baby's hour of need. It turned out that his bluff was never called, because the baby survived emergency treatment for an incarcerated hernia and got well.

When July first came along, Lester Martin had at last finished his nine years of surgical training. He was packing his belongings when Dr. Gross summoned him to his office. Dr. Marshal Lee had just submitted his resignation as Chief of Surgery at the Cincinnati Children's Hospital. If Lester would start at once, the job was his. This was one of the very best children's hospitals in the country. The fact that Lester could go straight from a residency to head the surgery department of so fine an institution was a tribute to him, of course, and we were overjoyed for him. But it made us all proud of ourselves as well, because we knew we were part of the finest pediatric surgical training program in the world.

11

Neurosurgery

When I reported for my first day of duty on neurosurgery I realized that in the sixteen months I had been at Children's Hospital I had never set foot on the neurosurgical floor. I was sure I would never put to use anything I was about to learn, since I had no intention of becoming a neurosurgeon, and I was convinced that in being made to work there for two months I was being shamefully exploited. I knew absolutely nothing about neurosurgery and was certain I was not going to like it. I was in for a very pleasant surprise.

Pediatric neurosurgery is almost exclusively an attack on the three great child-killers, injury, cancer, and congenital malformations. The ward contained forty of the sickest children I had ever seen. It took me only a few minutes to see why I, or somebody like me, was needed. The work load was prodigious. The lone neurosurgical resident spent many sixteen-hour days in the operating room, leaving me to provide all the supportive care these critically ill children required. Fortunately, the nurses were very knowledgeable and supremely helpful. Without them my job would have been impossible. Probably never in my whole training experience did I learn so much so fast. The two staff neurosurgeons, Dr. Matson and Dr. Ingraham, had just published a textbook detailing the conditions that brought children to them. That book was a godsend. I read it from cover to cover during the first week.

The neurosurgical resident was an ever-cheerful, chronically exhausted fellow named Walter Cotter. On early rounds, which started at five-thirty in the morning, and during the late evening hours after the operating schedule was finally finished, he taught me how to perform a neurological examination, a ritual that suddenly had much more meaning than when I had been briefly exposed to it in medical school. I soon found that with his teaching, and with the book and the nurses to lean on, I could figure out what was wrong with most of the patients when they came to the hospital and could predict fairly accurately what lay in store for them. This was especially important on the neurosurgical ward because Dr. Ingraham insisted that there be absolutely no visiting. I thought he carried it to an unnecessary extreme, but clearly some limitation of visiting was essential if the tremendous amount of work was going to get done. The parents brought their children to the ward, answered all the questions I could think of to ask them, and left. Even if their children were on the ward for a month or more, as many were, they never saw them again until the day they were discharged. I was the only link between children and parents, and my contacts with the parents were entirely over the phone.

After a month or six weeks of constant reassurance via long distance I am sure many parents built up mental pictures of intellectual improvement that contrasted bitterly with the reality they discovered when at last they came to take their poor little children home. Brain surgery doesn't add anything. It is essentially the art of removing as little as possible. Children have remarkable powers of recovery, especially when compared to those of adults, but even infants cannot grow a single new brain cell to replace one which has been destroyed or removed. Many children left the ward severely and permanently handicapped. Once the parents admitted to themselves that their children would never be completely normal again, the great majority faced this heartbreaking reality with a degree of courage I found tremendously inspiring. I came to know many people who were braver than I would have been had I faced similar burdens.

Jonas Salk was on the verge of perfecting the vaccine that would put an end to poliomyelitis, but there were as many polio cases that summer as in any average year. Many children with symptoms suggestive of brain tumors came to the neurosurgeons only to find that they had polio instead. Unfortunately, the reverse was also true. We worked closely with the pediatricians in sorting out these often puzzling cases, though we did not look after the children who actually had polio.

One afternoon Walter sent me down to examine a little boy in the emergency room. The mother left him alone with me while she went off to get a friend to look after her three other children. He was a sweet little child with big blue eyes. He had no fever, which was unusual for early polio, though it certainly did not rule out this diagnosis. He had a strange pattern of weakness, some muscles being almost totally paralyzed while others supplied by the same nerve groups seemed not at all affected. I could think of no brain tumor that would produce this spotty distribution of weakness and was about to conclude that the boy must have polio after all, when I accidentally discovered that he couldn't see. He was too young to read a regular eye chart, but only a few minutes before he had recognized the objects on the special chart we used for young children. He had gone completely blind, right before my eyes. If blindness were a part of his illness, it couldn't be polio. Cruel as polio was, it never inflicted blindness on its victims. The only disorder I could think of to explain what I found was multiple sclerosis, and that, I thought, was a disease that affected only adults. Walter's instructions had been to admit the boy to neurosurgery unless he had polio, so despite the fact that multiple sclerosis was not a surgical disease, that was what I did.

I never dreaded facing a mother as much as I did this one. Somehow, telling her that her little boy was blind seemed harder than it would have been to tell her he was going to die. I was mentally prepared for almost any reaction but the one I found. She accepted the news with no more emotion than if I had told her he needed a haircut. She was not cold or otherwise indifferent, and she appeared to love her little boy with all her heart. Perhaps there was a psychiatric explanation, some mental block put there by the benevolence of Nature to protect her from an unbearable pain. I've often wondered, but it remains one of the most amazing mysteries I ever witnessed.

When Walter finally got out of the operating room he

couldn't believe I had been so dumb as to admit so obvious a medical case to neurosurgery. Besides, how could my diagnosis of multiple sclerosis possibly be correct, since everyone knew it affected only adults? The pediatric residents couldn't believe it either when they came gleefully to collect him and take him to their ward. I was the butt of many a joke about how much a perfectly sensible pediatrician could forget if he allowed himself to associate with surgeons.

Next day the boy was presented at Grand Rounds, and Walter insisted that I attend as I obviously had much to learn. I slunk as unobtrusively as possible into a seat in the back row, consoling myself with the thought that Walter was probably secretly feeling guilty that he failed to notice that the boy was blind.

The case had been selected for presentation because a distinguished neurologist was visiting the hospital. The pediatric resident spared no detail in describing how admission to the proper service had been delayed by a neurosurgeon who had come up with the absurd diagnosis of multiple sclerosis.

"But," said the distinguished visitor, "multiple sclerosis does, in rare instances, affect children. That is exactly what this little boy has." A pin dropping in that hushed auditorium would have resounded like a crowbar falling into an empty garbage can. Walter never got over it.

One of the common problems we dealt with was hydrocephalus. Otherwise known as "water on the brain," this distressing problem resulted from delay in absorbing spinal fluid, most of which is actually not formed in the spinal canal but in the ventricles, or hollow spaces within the brain. There were two forms of hydrocephalus, known as the communicating and the non-communicating types. In the non-communicating form a congenital malformation blocked the narrow passage through which the fluid drained down to the spinal canal where normally most of it was absorbed. These infants were managed by placing a tube in the ventricle and using it to conduct the fluid to the abdominal cavity from which it was absorbed in a pretty satisfactory fashion. Dr. Matson had solicited the aid of a group of engineers at the Massachusetts Institute of Technology, and together they were developing an ingenious one-way valve, some form of which was essential to prevent backflow. There were all sorts of problems in keeping protein in the spinal fluid from coagulating and plugging up these delicate little valves. Dr. Matson spent many hours operating on these babies over and over again to replace obstructed valves. In another part of the country an engineer named Holter, whose own child had hydrocephalus, was simultaneously developing a somewhat larger but more reliable valve, and after I left the service, the Holter valve became the standard treatment for a while.

Children with the communicating form had a different problem. Here there was no obstruction in the brain itself, but an inability of the lining of the spinal canal to absorb the fluid at a normal rate. For them the treatment was simpler and more reliable since a valve was not required. A little tube was placed in the lower end of the spinal canal and led through the flank to the top of the ureter. The ureter is the tubular structure which conducts urine from the kidney to the bladder, and it normally has a downward propulsive action that prevents backflow. The operative results of this procedure were quite satisfactory, and reoperation was not very often required. The only drawback was that it was necessary to remove a kidney in order to use its ureter.

Part of my job was explaining to parents why this seemingly drastic procedure was necessary. I sat with one young mother for an hour or more late one afternoon going over the proposed operation. Sensing that she did not quite understand it, I suggested that she get some supper and return for another session. About eight o'clock she returned and I went over it all again. She listened intently as I explained that she was one of the luckier ones because her baby had the form of hydrocephalus for which we had the best operation. The spinal fluid in her baby's case was not trapped in the brain but could make its way to the spinal canal where we could drain it off by simply putting in a tube to lead it to the ureter. To do this we would have to remove one of her baby's kidneys so that we could use the ureter to drain the excess fluid. The baby would still have one normal kidney, which was all she would ever need. I thought my explanation had been particularly lucid, and I was quite taken aback when she gazed sorrowfully at her sleeping infant and sighed,

"Poor dear, so young to lose a lung!" Even when you tried really hard, you sometimes didn't get through.

Walter assigned me to assist Dr. Matson with the little baby's operation. Dr. Matson made the first incision and slipped the slender tube into the spinal canal. Then to my great surprise he put the knife in my hand and guided me through the major part of the operation, taking out the kidney and introducing the other end of the tube into the ureter. It was by far the most major operation I had ever been allowed to do, and it seemed ironic that this great privilege was given me by the man I had been so sure had been intent on exploiting me. Dr. Matson was a superb teacher and made me do every part of the procedure according to his exacting standards. It was the first of a number of very satisfying experiences I had with him. The baby did well and in a few days went home with her mother, who probably still has not the slightest idea what really happened to her little girl.

The next night, shortly after midnight, I got a call from Dr. Merritt Low in Greenfield, Massachusetts. When I had been in boarding school at Eaglebrook, in nearby Deerfield, Dr. Low had been my school doctor. He sounded relieved to be reaching a familiar voice so late at night. He told me he had a little girl who he was sure had a brain tumor, and he wanted to send her to Boston right away. I told him I would be on the lookout for her, and we reminisced briefly about the good old days when I had been one of his school boys.

She arrived about two hours later, and though she was drowsy and confused I couldn't see what the emergency was. I took the history from her anxious father, and we agreed that Dr. Low was a wonderful doctor. I assured him that we would take care of her as solicitously as Dr. Low had done and that I would be on the phone every night to give him a progress report. We shook hands and he went home, assuring me that he would call me every night. I put the little girl to bed and went to sleep myself, still wondering what had made Dr. Low consider it such an emergency.

Next morning Walter took one look at her and rushed her to the operating room. She had a pineal glioma, a tumor so precisely positioned that it would have killed her in a few more hours had the pressure it was causing not been relieved. The damage caused by the tumor and the operation needed to remove it was tremendous, and for several days she was little more than a vegetable. Slowly she began to awaken, and by the end of two weeks could remember her name. This she shouted incessantly at the top of her lungs. Whenever I asked her why she felt she had to shout she would scream, "I don't know!" If I close my eyes and listen I can hear her senseless screaming even now.

Her father never missed a night on the telephone. He was pathetically eager for any evidence of progress, and I was just as eager to find something reassuring but truthful to tell him. Finally, after four weeks, she could hold a spoon in her hand, though she had no idea what to do with it. Her father was overjoyed. For the life of me, I couldn't understand why he couldn't grasp how terribly damaged she was.

Years later my own father fell down a flight of stairs and spent four days in a coma in the intensive care unit of our local hospital. When he began to awaken, I would spend a few moments with him each evening before taking my mother home for the night. Every day he seemed to improve, until in our hopeful minds he seemed to have gone right past perfect. When he finally put on his clothes and came home from the foreign environment of the hospital we were amazed to see how far from perfect he really was. Fortunately, he went on to a full recovery, in sad contrast to this father's little girl. I chanced to meet him shortly thereafter and he told me how wonderfully she was progressing. He insisted that I come with him to his car to see her. She was a helpless imbecile. For the first time, I realized that I understood him.

On the hottest day of the summer good old Walter covered for me so I could hurry down the street to the Boston Lying-In Hospital for the birth of our fourth baby. I wore my hospital whites and tried to look nonchalant, but I don't think I fooled anybody. I was just as excited a new father as I had been when Jeff, Kate, or Amy had been born. In those days nobody held long debates about whether or not to have babies. Everyone who could had lots of them. Patty quite naturally expected her first three to be normal, and was happy but not particularly surprised when they were. This time, while awaiting the birth of her fourth, she had found time to volunteer once a week in a clinic filled with children with hare lips, cleft palates, and other birth defects. Try as she might to remember the odds against having a deformed baby, she couldn't totally repress the possibility. When Peter presented himself, normal in every way, her relief was enormous.

My rotation on neurosurgery ended while Patty and Peter were still in the hospital. Dr. Matson and Dr. Ingraham had been generous, kind, and considerate, and they and Walter had taught me a great deal that would be useful to me in the future. I was truly sorry to be leaving their service. As a final act of kindness Dr. Ingraham arranged for our membership in the Boston Skating Club. Here for three winters we and our three older children enjoyed many happy hours together. Here we watched the beautiful Olympic skating champion Tenley Albright, who had become a Harvard medical student, teach her tiny daughter to skate.

Peter came home to occupy the little room I had fixed up as a study but had never studied in. It was a tiny space, no more than six feet by eight, but it was perfect for a new baby. Before he outgrew it we would be moving West, though we had no inkling of this at the time.

12

Heart Surgery

In 1938 two surgeons, both in Boston, successfully ligated a patent ductus arteriosus. Dr. Strieder, who did it first, saw his patient safely to the recovery room but lost him in a tragic postoperative accident. Dr. Gross' patient lived. The era of modern heart surgery had begun.

The ductus arteriosus is a vessel less than half an inch long that runs between the aorta and the pulmonary artery. A patent ductus is one that remains open after it should have closed. The aorta distributes blood from the heart's powerful left ventricle to arteries that carry it to all parts of the body. After supplying the tissues with oxygen the blood returns to the heart and is pumped by the weaker right ventricle through the pulmonary artery to the lungs. Normally there is no way for blood to pass from one of these great vessels to the other after birth, but before birth this would be very unsatisfactory because the infant's unused lungs cannot accommodate all of the blood the heart delivers to the pulmonary artery. In order to bypass the unborn baby's lungs, part of this blood is shunted through the ductus arteriosus from the pulmonary artery to the aorta.

When the baby's lungs begin to expand at birth, resistance to blood flow through them is lowered dramatically and the pressure in the pulmonary artery falls to a tiny fraction of that in the aorta. If the ductus does not close spontaneously as it normally would at this time, the direction of blood flow through it reverses, causing blood which already has picked up a full load of oxygen in the lungs to be shunted back to them again. At first this is merely inefficient. To do its job the heart simply works harder than it should. Only the most astute parents notice that their child is having difficulty in keeping up with his peers. There are no other symptoms. The fact that the ductus has failed to close is discovered during a routine physical examination when a physician hears the machinery-like murmur made by blood rushing through the open ductus. If the ductus is then closed surgically the child goes on to live a normal life.

If the ductus is not closed in early childhood an insidious chain of events is set in motion which eventually dooms the child to die whether or not the ductus is closed later. The delicate blood vessels in the lungs, subjected day after day to the relentless pounding of blood forced through the open ductus, begin to constrict. As they do, they drive up the pressure in the pulmonary artery. When this pressure reaches and finally exceeds the pressure in the aorta the direction of the flow through the ductus again reverses, allowing some of the blood in the pulmonary artery to enter the aorta without picking up fresh oxygen in the lungs. As more and more blood is shunted away from the lungs the child becomes progressively oxygen-starved until he can no longer survive. Meanwhile, the ductus has begun to function as a safety valve for the overburdened right ventricle, and if a surgeon now attempts to close it, the heart promptly fails. A problem once easily correctable has become insoluble.

The first operations involved simply tying a ligature around the ductus, but it soon became apparent that to occlude the vessel permanently it is necessary to dissect it out very carefully, divide it between clamps, and oversew the ends with fine silk. In essence, the operation is very simple.

Not satisfied with having scored this historic first, Dr. Gross began at once to devise an attack on coarctation of the aorta. Though its cause is not known, coarctation is an easy abnormality to understand. It is simply an abrupt constriction in the aorta, usually at or very near the point of attachment of the ductus. Viewed from inside the aorta, it resembles a diaphragm with a pinhole in the center. The major arteries that supply the head and arms come off the aorta above the coarctation. Those supplying the body and legs come off below it. The diagnosis is easy to make if a physician takes the trouble to compare the pulses or measure the blood pressure in the arms and legs. The pressure in the arms is abnormally high, that in the legs immeasurably low. Like children with patent ductus, those with coarctation have few symptoms, but the tremendous burden on the heart severely shortens their life expectancy if the coarctation is not removed.

In 1944 Dr. Gross in Boston and Dr. Crafoord in Europe successfully removed coarctations for the first time. The operation consists of dissecting the narrowed segment free from surrounding structures, placing a special clamp on each side of it, removing it, and sewing the ends of the aorta together. When Dr. Gross did the operation it usually took him between two and five hours, depending on the age of the patient. It was not easy work, but many other operations are as demanding. Once they had seen it, cardiologists could not believe it had not been done years earlier. Another group of children with previously untreatable congenital heart disease could now be cured.

These two operations, together with the laboratory work that went into developing them, nearly won the Nobel Prize in Medicine for Dr. Gross. They were spectacular achievements, classically simple in concept and very effective. Far more ingenious, at least to my mind, was the method Dr. Gross developed to allow him to open a beating heart and close an interatrial septal defect.

Leading into the ventricles, which are the main pumping chambers of the heart, are two less powerful chambers called atria. Like the ventricles, the atria are separated from one another by a common wall called a septum. Before birth there are large openings in the interatrial septum which, like the patent ductus, allow some of the blood returning from the body to bypass the lungs. Persistence of a large opening after birth permits shunting that is no longer in the child's best interest. A little leakage is well tolerated, but a large defect is a serious handicap.

To permit him to close interatrial septal defects, Dr. Gross developed a device known as an atrial well. This was made of soft rubber like that used in surgeons' gloves. It was fashioned in the shape of a cone with the bottom cut off. The top was about eight inches in diameter and the opening at the bottom about two inches across. The lower edge had a reinforced margin so that it could be sutured securely to the outside of the atrial wall. When this had been done Dr. Gross made an incision in the wall of the heart at the bottom of the well. Blood immediately rushed out into the well, but the patient did not bleed to death. Instead, the outflow of blood stopped when the well was about three quarters full, and though the heart kept on beating, no further blood loss occurred. The column of blood in the well had risen as high as the pressure in the atrium would push it. Working blindly in a pool of blood three to four inches deep, Dr. Gross could introduce his finger into the atrium of the beating heart, and using this finger to guide his needle holder could place a row of sutures across the hole in the wall between the atria. Then he tied the sutures one by one, cut them with his finger guiding the long scissors, and, again solely by feel, sutured up the opening he had made in the wall of the heart.

The results with the atrial well were not as uniformly good as those of operations for patent ductus and coarctation because after the heart was opened some of the defects were found to be too large to close by pulling their edges together with sutures. These would have to wait, as did defects in the wall between the ventricles, for the day when the heart could be stopped and the defect attacked under direct vision, using synthetic material as a patch if necessary. In its day however, the atrial well provided an answer for some children for whom there never had been an answer before, and though it is no longer used, it still stands as a monument to a very ingenious mind.

One day an eager young cardiologist from Johns Hopkins named Helen Taussig sat in Dr. Gross' office and told him how to do an operation for "blue babies." She admitted that the operation she proposed had never been done, but she was sure it would work. Dr. Gross was not so sure and refused to try it. Another historic first had been handed to him on a silver platter, but he declined it. Dr. Taussig returned to Baltimore where Dr. Alfred Blalock proved more receptive. Her idea worked.

"Blue babies" have a relatively complicated malformation named for a French physician, Dr. Fallot. Since there are technically four parts to the anomaly, the disorder is known as the tetralogy of Fallot. The essence of the problem is that too little blood makes its way through an abnormally narrow inlet to the pulmonary artery, while too much of it makes its way through an interventricular septal defect to the aorta without going through the lungs at all. Circulation of poorly oxygenated blood gives the children a deep blue color known as cyanosis. Their exercise tolerance is severely limited and their life-span greatly shortened.

The ideal way to deal with the problem would be to close the interventricular septal defect and widen the narrow channel leading to the pulmonary artery. This can now be done, but at that time it was impossible. Dr. Taussig's simple solution was to divide the artery leading to the left arm and suture the end of it nearest the heart to the side of the pulmonary artery. This fell far short of correcting the anatomic abnormality, but it allowed more blood to reach the lungs and the children usually were greatly improved. Although the main channel to the arm was sacrificed there were plenty of smaller arteries to carry blood to the arm and hand.

Shortly after Dr. Blalock performed the operation Dr. Taussig had suggested, Dr. Willis Potts in Chicago devised a clever set of clamps that allowed him to suture the aorta and the pulmonary artery together, creating an artificial shunt for these deeply cyanotic children. These two procedures accomplished the same goal, palliation rather than cure.

A small group of children had pulmonic stenosis, the narrowing of the channel leading to the pulmonary artery, without the other features of tetralogy of Fallot. They were not blue, but their right ventricles had to work against tremendous resistance and their life expectancy was greatly reduced. Dr. Holmes Sellors in England devised a series of cutting devices that could be introduced through a small slit in the wall of the heart to enlarge the narrow channel.

These six operations—closure of patent ductus, removal of coarctation, closure of some interatrial septal defects using the atrial well, Dr. Blalock's and Dr. Potts' operations for tetralogy of Fallot, and widening the narrow channel of pulmonic stenosis—were the entire armamentarium of surgeons dealing with congenital heart defects in 1955.

Although closure of patent ductus and removal of coarctation of the aorta had ushered in the modern age of heart surgery, they were not operations on the heart itself. Neither were Dr. Blalock's nor Dr. Potts' operations for "blue babies." Dr. Sellors' cleverly designed cutting instruments and Dr. Gross' ingenious atrial well permitted abnormalities within the heart to be approached, but the surgeon had to work blindly, guided only by the clarity with which he could see the hidden defect in his mind's eye and feel it with his instruments or fingers. In addition, his target was constantly in motion. Major advances beyond these brilliant but limited beginnings had to await the development of a machine that could take over the functions of the heart and lungs, allowing the surgeon to stop the heart, open it, and empty it of blood so that he could deal with a motionless defect that he could clearly see.

There were several problems to overcome. Whenever a mechanical pump was used it was necessary to use something to keep the blood from clotting. This was the easiest part. The anticoagulant heparin had been well known for years. Its action was very predictable and easily reversed when no longer needed. Another problem with pumps was that they tended to be physically damaging to blood cells. The earliest models could be used for only a few minutes before the damage became prohibitive. This problem was gradually overcome by milking the blood through plastic tubing compressed by a series of mechanical fingers or rollers so that the blood never came in contact with the pump's moving parts. Several investigators developed pumps that could be used for an hour or more, which would be ample time to repair most of the intracardiac defects known to exist.

Regardless of the safety and efficacy of a pump, it was useless if the blood it circulated was not rich in oxygen. The most difficult problem was how to add oxygen to the blood and remove carbon dioxide from it. A pump by itself could not perform these functions, nor had a pump been devised that could allow the patient's lungs to do their usual work while the heart was stopped. Two types of oxygenators proved about equally effective. In one the blood was pumped through a long channel made of a special plastic membrane which was surrounded by oxygen. The pores in the membrane were just the right size to allow oxygen to flow into the blood and carbon dioxide to escape. As it flowed from one end of the tube to the other, one could see the dark blood change to bright red as its oxygen content increased.

The second approach involved using a series of rotating discs to expose a thin film of blood directly to oxygen. The blood was pumped into the bottom of a glass pipe about four inches in diameter which lay on its side. Less than a quarter of the pipe was filled with blood; the remainder was filled with oxygen. A series of vertical discs like small phonograph records rotated in the pipe, their edges dipping down into the blood and carrying a thin film of it up into the oxygen and back down again to the pool of blood beneath. As the blood moved slowly beneath this series of discs from one end of the pipe to the other it became a brighter and brighter red. From the far end of the pipe it was gathered and pumped to the patient.

Dr. Gross chose the disc oxygenator and spent many hours in the laboratory working out the details of its use. Before I joined his service he had used his pump-oxygenator, which came to be known simply as the "pump," on twelve children. Nine of them had died. Three had lived. The nine who died certainly died when they did because they had been subjected to operations that didn't work, but all twelve had such serious heart defects that none could have been expected to live very long had nothing been done for them. They had been carefully selected patients for whom no operation without the use of the "pump" could possibly have been beneficial. The death toll of this first trial was horrendous, but compared to the alternative, the salvage of 25 percent was a spectacular achievement. Many advances in surgery have been made by raising the outlook from hopeless to poor and going on from there, but it takes tremendous courage to persist after having to tell nine sets of parents that your efforts have failed to save their children. After a year of further work in the laboratory Dr. Gross brought an improved "pump" back to the operating room. This time the results were very much better.

It was during this hiatus, while the "pump" was back in the laboratory, that Tom Holder and I served as senior and junior resident on Dr. Gross' service. Tom had been halfway through his chief residency in a general surgery program when a chance to fit into Dr. Gross' senior residency had arisen. His department chairman had such high regard for Tom that he let him go away to Boston for two years and held the final six months of his chief residency open for him. If anyone deserved such extraordinary consideration, Tom certainly did. His distinguished career in Kansas City, which included the presidency of the American Pediatric Surgical Association, came as no surprise to anyone who knew him as a resident.

Summer is a busy time for pediatric surgeons because children are not in school. Children of school age who need elective operations tend to wait until school is out to have them done. Few girls mention it, but many a boy has assured me that waiting until summer was his parents' idea, not his. The cardiac operations usually fell into the elective category; that is, operations that were not emergencies and could be scheduled at the convenience of the parents or the surgeon. Dr. Gross had a sizable backlog of operations for ductus and coarctation, and we often did two or three in a day. It was the most concentrated exposure to major operations I ever experienced in my training, and I never had a two-month period in my own practice to match it.

Patients with coarctation came to Dr. Gross from all over the world. The ideal age for the operation was felt to be between four and ten years, but there were many patients who had grown past this optimal age, and though he limited his surgery almost entirely to children, Dr. Gross did accept adult patients with coarctation. During my first week one of the most beautiful girls I had ever seen came to Dr. Gross from Paris. Tom and I were the envy of all our colleagues, and we felt justly so. On the day before her operation a group of French cardiologists came with us on rounds, accompanied by one of our nurses who spoke some halting French. I have never forgotten the look of amazement on the face of one of them when he recognized this lovely creature as his patient. He had referred her to Dr. Crafoord, but she had chosen, unbeknownst to him, to come to Dr. Gross instead. She was mortified to have been discovered, and he made every effort to assure her that he was not offended, though dismay was written all over his face. I had not admitted it for fear of being given the role of interpreter, but I knew enough French to take in their conversation. As soon as the visitors were out of earshot I repeated it for Tom and Dr. Gross and we howled with laughter. I have often wondered if any other residents have seen Dr. Gross enjoy so hearty a laugh. It was a rare crack in his icy reserve. The next morning the whole French group crowded into the gallery and watched through the roof of the glass enclosure as Dr. Gross performed the most technically perfect operation they, or I, had ever seen.

Not all of the operations ended as happily as that one. We took a little girl to the operating room one morning expecting to find a small interatrial septal defect only to discover that the hole was so huge that the edges could not be brought together. The unsuccessful operation was more than her overworked heart could stand. She lived only a couple of hours.

As is often the case, the little girl's mother was far better prepared for bad news than her husband. She knew better than he the hopelessness of her daughter's outlook had this effort not been made and instinctively knew that they had made the best decision for her in permitting the operation to go forward. He had heard the same warnings from Dr. Gross that his wife had, but had let them go in one ear and out the other. He could not accept defeat. I gently suggested that they might like to see their little girl. As I knew they would, she declined and he accepted. I led him along the corridor to the operating room. There she lay, unconscious and barely breathing, surrounded by every device a modern operating room could contain. As he approached his beloved little girl it finally hit him.

"Isn't there anything more you can do?" he whispered, and then without waiting for a reply he added, "No, I can see there isn't." He bent over her tiny form and kissed her forehead. Her eyes were closed, but the look on her face was the serene look little girls get when they dream pleasant dreams. He followed me numbly back to his wife and they wept quietly together. As I turned to leave he clutched my hand and said almost inaudibly, "Please thank Dr. Gross for both of us."

When I returned to the operating room she had stopped breathing. I silently thanked this little girl for living long enough for her father to see her. It had been almost unbearably painful for him, but it had done for him what no words could possibly have accomplished. There would be no doubts to haunt him. He had seen for himself that nothing that could have been done to save his daughter had been omitted. He could live with that.

The next day Leopold, former King of the Belgians, and his princess, Lillian, brought their son Alexander to Dr. Gross with a coarctation. During World War II the king had kept his country out of the fighting, sparing it the devastation that surely would have rained down upon it had he done otherwise. His people had been ambivalent about this decision, and when peace returned to Europe, Leopold had abdicated in favor of his son Baudouin. Leopold's queen had been killed in an automobile accident, and he had married Lillian, who had been engaged to supervise his children's education. It was their son, King Baudouin's younger half brother, who came to Boston.

The hospital responded in a manner fit in every way for royalty. An entire floor, previously unused, was opened for them in the new wing of the hospital. There was a sizable retinue. Several Belgian equivalents of our Secret Service men occupied the rooms nearest the elevators. Lillian took up residence in the room next to that of her son and used the room across the hall as a sitting room. A couple of maids had the room beyond his. Leopold and another group of civil servants lived in a nearby hotel. Tom and I were the only house officers permitted on the floor and were the center of attention at the peanut-butter-and-jelly sessions. I had fully expected to be displaced by one of the seniors, but I wasn't.

Every time the young prince left his room I went with him. We spent an hour in the X-ray Department and half an hour in the EKG lab. The next day we went to Dr. Nadas' office where the prince was examined as if his diagnosis were a deep mystery, his x-rays and electrocardiogram studied as if those he had brought with him from the leading cardiologist in Belgium had been lost in the Atlantic Ocean. The inevitable diagnosis was reached, and Dr. Nadas explained the condition to Lillian as if she did not already know from her own physician and from her reading almost everything there was to know about coarctation. It seemed superfluous, but of course it wasn't. There could be no surprises when a prince went into the operating room.

Every possible contraindication to operating on the prince was looked for. None was found, but the screening process took longer than usual, and the boy was in the hospital for nearly a week before his operation was scheduled. I got to know him and his mother very well during that week. He spoke English slowly, with long pauses as he groped for the correct word, but he made himself understood more readily than he realized. He was very bright but painfully shy. I know I understood his conversation better than he understood mine as I am sure I used words he had never heard before. I tried to explain each procedure to him before he encountered it, but I knew that he was accepting a great deal on faith. His mother spoke several languages fluently, including French, Spanish, German, and English. She was a beautiful woman, considerably younger than the king, and she openly thought Dr. Gross was wonderful. He wasn't very good at hiding his admiration for her either.

The operation began as routinely as any other. The gallery was filled with Belgian physicians, with Dr. Nadas at their elbow to explain what was going on. Unlike Lillian, they understood almost no English, especially English with a Hungarian accent. However much they may have missed of the description, they were suitably dazzled by what they saw.

Wide exposure is essential in removing a coarctation. Dr. Gross made a generous incision in the left side of the young prince's chest. Almost at once he started hunching his shoulders, a sure sign that he was displeased. We worked in total silence for a while, and then Dr. Gross put down his instrument and suggested in a loud voice that Dr. Nadas might like to take the doctors to reassure Lillian that everything was going smoothly. They rose in unison and departed. As soon as the door to the gallery closed behind them he enlarged the incision by a generous three inches and the shoulder-hunching stopped. When they returned everything was going like clockwork.

Despite all reassurances, the prince had been very frightened of the operation. His adult conversation and the deference shown him by everyone had made it easy to forget that he was only fourteen years old. When he awoke he seemed totally disoriented, as if he had expected to wake from a dream in his familiar bedroom far across the ocean. His convalescence was otherwise uneventful, but I was so caught up in expecting a prince to progress faster than a mere mortal that I felt it was unusually slow. Of course he had to stay in the hospital longer than if he were going home to a suburb of Boston.

He was barely able to sit up when the lesson books reappeared. I suggested gently to his mother that perhaps his schooling was being resumed prematurely, but was treated to a look that told me in no uncertain terms how little I knew about princes.

On Sunday, some five days after the operation, he was allowed out of bed for three or four hours, and Lillian let it be known that the prince loved to play the piano. Nobody seemed to know where a piano might be found on Sunday. I was sent in search of one.

In an older part of the hospital I finally located one in a playroom filled with toys for children of all ages. The playroom was never used unless an authorized "play lady" was there to supervise the children, and on Sunday it was locked up tighter than a drum. I eventually gained access to it by crawling in through a dumb waiter. After I discovered that the door could be unlocked from the inside and that the room could be made private by closing the curtains on all the windows that gave on the corridor, I phoned his nurse and told her to wheel the prince over for his piano recital.

I waited for an eternity, peeking out through a crack in the curtains at the faces of children who were assuring their parents that it was okay to play in the playroom as long as someone from the hospital was there. They were pretty sure someone was. I tried a few notes on the ancient piano, which was badly out of tune. Now they were all certain that someone was inside. I was fast losing what little enthusiasm I had brought to the project when the prearranged series of knocks signaled the arrival of the prince.

He eased himself out of his wheelchair onto the hard piano bench with the look of a child facing a bowl of tepid spinach and began a simple piece which he played very badly. It was obvious that in addition to his lack of enthusiasm and limited musical ability it hurt him to move his left arm. The brief recital came to a merciful end, but not before his nurse had taken the opportunity to apologize profusely for keeping me waiting so long. As soon as the prince had gotten word of the impending encounter with the piano he had gone into hiding, and it had taken her nearly an hour to find him.

At last the great day arrived when the prince was to be discharged. He would spend a week or ten days in a nearby hotel before flying home to Belgium. The packing and repacking seemed endless. Tom and I waited with Dr. Gross to say our farewells. There were two things Dr. Gross hated. One was being kept waiting. The other was having his picture taken. Today he was waiting to have his picture taken with the prince. The pained expression on his face was priceless.

To lessen Dr. Gross' discomfort I took the opportunity to tell him about a little boy with coarctation who had come up from Argentina the night before. Yes, Dr. Gross had been expecting him, what had delayed him? The father had remained in Argentina, sending the boy and his mother up alone. When they arrived in New York they both had such severe diarrhea that they had decided to spend the night in a hotel rather than endure the anguish of a ride on another plane to Boston. In the process the mother had used up all the money she had brought with her and the additional funds her husband was to have wired from Argentina had failed to arrive. Weak, exhausted, and temporarily penniless, they had straggled into the hospital at midnight. The mother spoke virtually no English, and had been reduced to near panic. She was utterly convinced that she was leading her son to slaughter.

Dr. Gross seemed strangely cheered by this news. For the first time in an hour he stopped hunching his shoulders. He turned on his heel and marched down the corridor toward the prince's suite. The procession had finally gotten in gear. Toward us came the king with his princess on his arm, the familiar pink slip in his hand indicating that his son had been cleared for discharge by the hospital cashier. Behind the king came the prince in his wheelchair, followed by the maids and civil servants carrying innumerable suitcases and bundles.

The king watched in speechless amazement as Dr. Gross

scooped the princess off his arm and announced, "Got a little job for you." The procession came to a halt and remained in frozen animation for almost ten minutes before the princess and Dr. Gross reappeared, both smiling broadly. In those ten minutes a frightened mother from Argentina had been reassured in her native tongue by the one person best qualified to reassure her, a mother whose own son had gone through the same dreaded operation and was now going home.

The procession resumed as if a stalled movie projector had been turned on again and we all made our way to the main lobby. Here instead of turning toward the front door we turned in the opposite direction and entered a little courtyard. The new wing of the hospital had closed off this little space, making it a barren quadrangle where the groundskeepers parked their lawnmowers. Almost overnight it had been transformed into a beautiful garden with flowering shrubs, paths, and inviting benches. This transformation, I learned, had been made possible through the generosity of Olive Higgins Prouty, author of *Stella Dallas*. What better way to acknowledge her generosity than to reveal the existence of the garden to the Boston press during the ceremonial discharge of a prince?

The photographs were endless. First the prince, standing by one of the benches. Then the king, Lillian, and Dr. Gross. Then the whole surgical team, including anesthetists and nurses. It went on and on. The prince was wan and tired before it was over. He sat down at every opportunity. In addition to the photographer, two reporters had wormed their way into the garden. I thought their restraint was admirable, but they did need a story. At one juncture they asked the prince if he would like to return when he was older and go to Harvard. He gave his charming smile and said that would be very nice. He was a pro at talking to reporters; he said nothing extra. Then he stood up for another picture. When he sat down again the reporters asked him the obvious question, "How do you feel so soon after your big operation?" By this time the prince was exhausted. "Very well," he replied weakly. Instantly realizing that he hadn't given this last answer his all, he added earnestly, "Very well, really, very well."

At last it was over. The procession entered the hospital and crossed the lobby to the waiting limousines. As the prince's wheelchair stopped at the front door Lillian bent down and whispered in his ear, "You should have said 'very well, thank you.'"

13

Hernias

Almost anything that followed two months with Tom Holder and Dr. Gross would have been anticlimactic, but my return to the chief resident's service did have two redeeming features. For the first time in all the months I had been at Children's Hospital I was not low man on the totem pole. We had a new "pup" to do the basic chores. In addition, my turn had come at last to do more than an occasional operation.

Lester Martin was gone, and we all missed him, but Bob Allen was a worthy successor as chief resident. He was somewhat less compulsive than Lester, which made it easier for him to delegate responsibility. He was keenly aware of the need for his junior residents to learn to operate and was constantly on the lookout for children with conditions suitable for us to operate upon. Among these were many babies and children with inguinal hernias.

Inguinal hernias are hernias in the groin. The typical hernias of childhood are very different from the "ruptures" that men and women acquire later in life. They are easier to correct and recurrences after repair are far less frequent. In his textbook Dr. Gross was able to report more than eight thousand operations for inguinal hernias in infants and children with only six recurrences, despite the fact that more than half of these operations had been done by junior residents like myself. Of course, a senior resident or staff surgeon participated in every operation as assistant and teacher.

It is estimated that one boy in twenty and one girl in two hundred is born with an inguinal hernia. These hernias are all present from birth, though some of them may not be detected for many months thereafter. Like many other developmental abnormalities they represent structures that were normal at one stage of growth but have persisted into a later stage wherein they are no longer normal.

The abdominal wall in the inguinal area consists of six layers: skin, fat, three layers of muscle, and peritoneum. The peritoneum is a moist shiny membrane about as thick as the wall of a child's toy balloon. It lines the abdominal cavity and extends over the stomach, intestines, liver, and spleen, preventing them from adhering to each other or to the body wall. The kidneys lie behind the peritoneum. In little boys the testicles are formed near the kidneys, high up in the retroperitoneal space. They gradually migrate downward and emerge through the muscle layers of the abdominal wall to enter the scrotum at about the time of birth. Every testicle must make this journey because the lower temperature in the scrotum is essential to production of fertile sperm. As a testicle descends it carries with it the artery that nourishes it, the vein that drains it, and the vas deferens that later will carry the sperm. These structures make up the spermatic cord.

The peritoneum facilitates this downward migration by giving rise to the processus vaginalis, a funnel-shaped sac of peritoneum that precedes the testicle into the scrotum. The testicle descends behind the processus and becomes enveloped in its lower portion. Normally, the part of the processus from the top of the testicle to the abdominal cavity becomes obliterated and persists in the spermatic cord as a fine fibrous strand. The hernia of childhood is a processus vaginalis that has not become obliterated.

In little girls the processus behaves in the same manner, emerging through identical openings in the muscle layers before becoming obliterated. Thus, all boys and all girls have hernias during part of their normal intrauterine life. If there is no testicle to descend behind the processus the sac begins to close somewhat earlier and is more likely to go on to complete obliteration. After birth the incidence of hernias in girls is only about one tenth that in boys.

If the openings in the muscle layers were situated directly in front of one another, the incidence of hernias would probably be much higher than it actually is. The resulting canal would be very short, and a loop of intestine could easily wedge its way out alongside the spermatic cord. To prevent the emergence of abdominal contents while providing a permanent exit for the cord, the openings are staggered. The opening in the inner muscle layer is above and lateral to that in the outer layer. In this way a canal is produced through which the cord runs downward and medially with the inner muscle layer behind it and the outer layer in front of it. In an adult this canal is about an inch and a half long. When the pressure within the abdomen rises, as during a sneeze, the muscles contract and temporarily reduce the space within the canal. It is said that at the peak of a sneeze the cord is so tightly compressed that blood flow through it stops momentarily.

The middle muscle layer gives rise to a long sleeve of muscle called the cremaster that surrounds the cord and follows the testicle to the scrotum. In little boys, whose testicles remain about the size of peanuts until puberty, contraction of the cremaster can pull the testicle up to the mouth of the canal where it may be hidden behind a thick layer of fat and may be thought by anxious parents, and even by an unwary physician, to be absent. This retraction is harmless, except for the anxiety it may cause, and when the testicle enlarges and becomes heavier in the early teen years the cremaster loses most of its retractile ability.

Some hernias are obvious when a baby is born, but the majority are not. Even if it is quite large, the peritoneal sac cannot be felt when it is empty since its walls are paper-thin. Only when something that belongs inside the abdomen enters the sac and distends it can one note a bulge in the groin. Usually the mother notices while bathing her child that the two sides of the groin area are not symmetrical. Sometimes this asymmetry is first noted by a pediatrician during a routine checkup.

The bulge is almost invariably caused by the presence in the sac of a loop of the baby's intestine. As long as this intestinal loop can slide easily back into the abdomen no harm is done, though some mothers report that their babies are less fussy and appear more comfortable after the hernia has been repaired than before. The reason hernias are dangerous is that the intestine may become incarcerated, or trapped. The walls of the canal may compress the intestine enough to produce engorgement of its veins and cause the portion outside the canal to become so swollen that it cannot return to the abdomen.

Incarceration is an emergency and is fatal if not relieved. Food cannot make its way through the trapped segment of intestine, and if the cycle of engorgement and swelling continues the bowel may die because of impaired circulation. In addition, the swollen intestine compresses the blood vessels of the testicle and may irreparably damage it.

The surprising thing is that incarceration, with all its attendant risks, occurs far more frequently in infants than in older children. I have heard many explanations to account for this, but never one that I thought was very plausible. It is simply a fact, but it is a very important fact because it means that the younger the baby is when the hernia is first discovered the more urgent it is to have it repaired promptly. Advising parents of tiny babies to wait until they are older, when presumably they will be better able to withstand an operation, is exactly the wrong advice to give them. Even in older children a hernia operation should not be unduly delayed, because incarceration can and does occur at any age.

The operation is basically very simple. The objective is to ligate and divide the sac at the point where it emerges from the abdomen and enters the inguinal canal. To do this the surgeon makes a short incision in the skin crease above the one that separates the abdomen from the leg. This crease is very prominent in babies and indicates the site where the scar will be least noticeable after the incision heals. After dividing the underlying fat the surgeon comes upon the outer of the three muscle layers. Upon dividing this layer he finds himself looking into the inguinal canal at the cremaster muscle fibers surrounding the spermatic cord. The hernia sac is contained within this muscular sleeve and is readily apparent when its fibers are teased apart. The vas deferens and blood vessels of the testicle are adherent to the sac and must be carefully separated from it before it is tied off and cut. It is not necessary to remove all of the sac as long as it is divided so that scar tissue can become interposed between the cut ends to prevent recanalization. Now the cord is replaced in its normal position and the wall of the canal sutured in front of it. Closure of the fat and skin completes the procedure. Often while the child is still asleep the same steps are repeated on the opposite side, even if there has been no evidence of a second hernia. About a third of children with one hernia will be found to have an open sac on the opposite side and may be spared a second operation by having it closed at this time.

The hernias found in little girls are just like those of little boys except that the inguinal canal does not contain a spermatic cord. Incarceration of intestine occurs in exactly the same way and presents the same degree of emergency. Occasionally a small, movable peanut-shaped mass can be felt in the hernia of a baby girl. This is the ovary. It may be present in the sac for some time without producing any discomfort or problem, but if incarceration of a loop of intestine occurs while the ovary is out in the sac the ovary may be destroyed by compression of its blood supply.

Despite our best efforts to avoid the complications of incarceration by operating on children soon after their hernias were discovered, a number of infants came to the emergency room with hernias already incarcerated. Sometimes the hernia had been recognized, and some had even had their operations scheduled, but many were not even suspected of having a hernia until incarceration had already occurred. The infants were very fussy and obviously in pain, partly because of the local discomfort and partly because they could not retain their feedings and were starving. Their mothers often did not know what the matter was, but they were invariably certain that something was seriously wrong with their babies. A glance at the inguinal region was all that was required to make the diagnosis. The biggest danger was that an unwary intern or resident would find a sore throat or red eardrum to account for the baby's distress and would send the baby home with a prescription before taking the diaper off.

Sometimes the incarcerated loop of intestine could not be returned to the abdomen, and we had to perform an emergency operation. This was never desirable because the operation was difficult and the hernia sac very liable to tear. Also the risk of anesthesia was greater, since the baby had intestinal obstruction and was likely to vomit and inhale regurgitated formula into his lungs. All operations are more risky when performed as emergencies than under elective conditions. Often there is no choice, but with incarcerated hernias there usually was. We put the babies to bed in little cribs with their feet higher than their heads. To keep them from rolling out of this position it was necessary to tie their feet securely to the foot of the crib with soft sheet wadding. We sedated them with Seconal or morphine and placed a tiny ice bag over the swelling in the groin. Then we waited for an arbitrary two-hour period. The exhausted baby usually dropped off to sleep, and in the head-down position the intestine often slipped into the abdomen of its own accord or could be gently coaxed in with our fingers after the muscles of the abdominal wall had been relaxed for a while. The hernia could then be repaired electively a day or two later. The two-hour time limit had been arrived at empirically, it being found that if the intestine would return to the abdomen without the need for an emergency operation it usually would do so within two hours. The incidence of gangrene of the intestine or testicle was not significantly increased unless this time limit was exceeded. The little baby whose physician had thrust him into my arms so that I would be the one the father killed had been treated in this way and had undergone an elective operation two days later.

14

Lucy

There is an old saying to the effect that there is no minor surgery, there are only minor surgeons. There is some truth to this, of course, because every operation is important and should be done with skill and care, but the slogan has survived for decades because of its ability to bolster the egos of surgeons when they experience a run of simple operations with nothing really major in sight. We all go through periods in our practices when it seems that every physician who refers us patients has forgotten our magnificent talents and will never again send us a child whose operation could not safely be turned over to a second-year medical student. While I was mastering the simple operations which make up the bulk of every pediatric surgeon's practice, Bob Allen was doing some very complex procedures. These seem to come in bunches, and while I was working for him Bob had a run of children with severe abnormalities of the esophagus. The most appealing of these was a little girl named Lucy.

Lucy was five years old when she let her curiosity get her into very deep trouble. She was playing in the basement of her home one day when she spotted a Coca-Cola bottle in a cleaning closet and took a generous swig from it. It was full of concentrated lye.

She was deathly ill but was kept alive with intravenous feedings until her esophagus began to heal. When she was first allowed to drink she seemed to handle liquids well enough, but as the weeks went by she began to have more and more trouble until she could force down only a few sips of water. When she was given a suspension of barium to swallow, the x-rays showed that a rigid sleeve of scar tissue encircled the injured portion of her esophagus, constricting it so tightly that only a narrow channel remained. The trickle of barium that made its way through this stricture was no wider than a piece of string.

Over the next two years Lucy was admitted seventeen times to Children's Hospital. On each admission she was taken to the operating room and put to sleep. Dilators, which looked like slender carrots with long stiff wire handles, were forced through her scarred esophagus, beginning with one barely wider than the wire itself and ending with one about a quarter of an inch wide. After each dilatation she was able to swallow normally for a few days, but within two or three weeks the old trouble always recurred. Once she returned to the hospital a few hours after a dilatation with shaking chills and a high fever. The dilator had perforated her esophagus.

Fortunately, the fever subsided without the need for drastic measures, but further dilatations were too dangerous to undertake. Lester Martin put in a gastrostomy tube, a rubber tube sewn into her stomach and brought out through an opening in her abdominal wall. Her mother found that nourishing Lucy through this gastrostomy tube was so much easier than trying to feed her by mouth that for a long time she refused to bring her back for any further treatment. When Bob finally convinced her to bring Lucy back she had nourished her entirely through this tube for more than a year.

Lucy was a little short for her age but her mother had fattened her up with all kinds of food put through a Waring blender and all other signs of starvation had disappeared. She had had so many unpleasant experiences in the hospital that she might well have been withdrawn and fearful, but she wasn't. She marched into the ward and made herself at home as if she had always lived there. When the "pup" told her he would have to start an intravenous infusion she put out her arm, made a fist and pointed to a vein in her forearm. "It always works when they put it here," she told him.

There were the usual conferences, and it was decided that Lucy needed a new esophagus. During one of these conferences

Dr. Gross asked her if she ever vomited. "I don't know how to vomit," she replied, as if he should have known. Everyone loved Lucy.

The history of esophageal replacement is a long and fascinating one. Among the first successful attempts was a series of operations to fashion a tube of skin taken from the chest and abdomen. When it was finally completed it bridged the gap between the throat and stomach, but it had many drawbacks more serious than the unsightly deformity it caused. The tube had no propulsive force and emptied only by gravity. There were many leaks, some of which took months to heal. The acid stomach juice was terribly corrosive to the skin that lined the tube, and whenever the tube leaked, the leaking area was greatly narrowed by scar tissue as it healed.

Others attempted to use a tube constructed of small intestine. The small intestine is of about the same diameter as the esophagus and does have propulsive force. The vessels supplying it are relatively short and limit the distance the upper end of the segment of intestine can be moved. If too many of these vessels are sacrificed in an attempt to gain length, the upper end of the substitute esophagus cannot survive. Sometimes the tube can be brought up a little farther by placing it upside down, but because of its natural propulsive action, food can only pass through it with great difficulty if the tube is oriented in the wrong direction. Most important is the fact that the small intestine, although much more resistant than the skin, is susceptible to ulceration when exposed for long periods to acid stomach juice. Some children with esophageal substitutes made of small intestine do reasonably well, but many are plagued with serious recurrent problems.

The best solution seemed to be to use a part of the colon. The colon is much wider than the normal esophagus and lacks the vigorous propulsive force of the small intestine, but it is very resistant to corrosion by stomach juice. The blood vessels that nourish it are often longer than those of the small intestine and are usually arranged in such a way that a long segment of colon can be brought up through the chest to the neck. A suture line between the real esophagus and the substitute is much easier to construct in the neck than in the chest, and if it leaks a little, as many of them do at first, the consequences are less dangerous. It was decided that Bob should provide Lucy with a new esophagus constructed from a piece of her colon. He dreaded having to tell her, but she accepted the news without protest.

We took Lucy to the operating room and the anesthetist put her to sleep. To sterilize the area in which we would be working, I painted her skin with iodine from the tip of her chin to the tops of her thighs. We were embarking on a major undertaking. We opened her abdomen through a long incision and inspected her colon. The colon begins at the end of the small intestine low on the right side of the abdomen, runs up along the right side, across to the left side above the umbilicus, and down the left side to the rectum. In adults the colon is about 3 feet long and 3 inches wide. Lucy's was proportionately smaller. We would have to use about half of it to construct a new esophagus. The immediate question was which half to use.

The artery leading to the midportion is relatively short, so whichever half of the colon is used, the end nearest the middle must remain in the abdomen while the other end, either the right where it joins the small intestine or the left where it joins the rectum, is the end that is brought up to the neck. It used to be thought that the right half would be preferable because food would travel through it from mouth to stomach in the direction that colon contents normally travel, whereas if the left half were used, food would have to go in the reverse direction, but we now know that this doesn't make much difference. The key to success lies in selecting the portion of colon with the most suitable blood supply.

The arteries that carry blood to the colon fan out from two short main trunks arising on the front of the aorta. As they travel to the colon the feeding arteries are linked together by vessels that run parallel to the colon, an arrangement reminiscent of that of a post-and-rail fence. Should one or more of the feeding vessels be interrupted, blood can still reach the colon by traveling through these connecting vessels. In order to move a segment of colon up through the chest to the neck, all but one of its main feeding vessels must be severed. The veins have a similar, though not identical arrangement. Both the arterial supply and the venous drainage must be adequate for the colon segment to survive.

Bob decided that the arrangement of vessels in the right half of Lucy's colon appeared suitable. He isolated all of the vessels he proposed to divide and put bulldog clamps across them. These are little clamps with bits of rubber protecting their tips. The pressure they exert is controlled by little springs so that they occlude the vessels without injuring them. When they were all in place the substitute esophagus was fed by a single artery and drained by a single vein.

Now we waited. The clock on the operating room wall ticked off the minutes. It seemed an eternity. After ten minutes the entire length of colon remained pink and healthy. Its muscle contracted vigorously when it was pinched with a forceps. The tiny vessels running over the colon wall still had pulsations that we could see and feel. It would be safe to proceed.

One by one we removed the bulldog clamps and tied and cut the feeding vessels. Next we divided the small intestine where it joined the colon so that every inch of the right half of the colon could be used. We divided the colon at its midpoint and sutured the remaining left half of the colon to the end of the small intestine, restoring continuity to the digestive tract. Lucy would have a few loose bowel movements at first but would soon adapt to her shortened colon. The substitute esophagus was as pink and healthy as before.

Now Bob made a short incision in Lucy's neck, and working from the neck downward and from the abdomen upward made a wide tunnel through her chest in front of her heart. I expected a lot of bleeding which would be hard to control in the depths of this tunnel, but there was none. He passed a long clamp down through the tunnel and pulled the end of the colon with the appendix still attached up in front of the liver into the tunnel and out through the incision in her neck. The colon segment had seemed very generous lying in the abdomen, but it barely made it through the tunnel and only the very tip of it emerged through the upper opening. Bob removed the appendix and sutured the end of the colon to the edges of the skin. We could still see pulsations in the tiny blood vessels. Nevertheless, the connection between the colon and the upper end of the esophagus would not be made until ten days later when all danger that the blood supply might fail had passed.

The next step was to make an opening in Lucy's stomach and suture the lower end of the new esophagus to it. To do this we had to take out the gastrostomy tube, but when the line of sutures was completed we put in a new one. Lucy would not swallow through her new esophagus for almost a month.

Bob let me close the long abdominal incision under his watchful eye, though he could have done it himself in half the time. I would close a lot of incisions other people had made before I did an operation of this magnitude myself.

Ten days later Lucy was back in the operating room. This time only the neck incision had to be reopened. I had expected that finding her scarred esophagus would be difficult, but Bob made it look easy enough, and the upper end of her colon segment was quickly sutured to it. The skin was closed over this suture line.

Lucy was up and running around the ward a few hours after this operation. The "pup" had to dive under a bed to catch her so he could start her intravenous at bed time. About two weeks later she went to the X-ray Department for a barium swallow which showed that her new esophagus filled and emptied without hesitation. That night there was a party on the ward. Lucy blew out eight candles and ate a piece of her birthday cake. It was the first mouthful of solid food she had swallowed in almost three years.

In addition to helping children with lye strictures there were other uses for colon interposition. Some children were born with malformations of the esophagus in which the two ends were so far apart that they could not be brought together. Every attempt was made to repair the esophagus because no substitute is as good as an esophagus itself, but it wasn't always possible. The babies had gastrostomy tubes put in at birth and were nourished through them for at least a year before the colon interposition was undertaken. Some had great difficulty in learning to swallow, having never done it before, but with patience they all could be taught to do so. For them, as for children with lye strictures, the colon made a very satisfactory substitute.

A third group for whom it was thought that a colon interposition might be helpful were children with esophageal varices. These are varicose veins lying just beneath the lining of the esophagus. They result from cirrhosis of the liver, a disorder I had thought affected only elderly alcoholics. Cirrhosis affects two groups of children, those with malformations of the bile ducts and those who survive severe attacks of neonatal hepatitis.

All of the blood returning from the digestive tract goes via the portal vein to the liver on its way to the heart. The liver filters out some of the nutrients which the blood has picked up from the intestine. Cirrhosis, or fibrotic scarring of the liver, impedes the passage of blood and raises the pressure in all of the veins leading to the portal vein. This increased pressure, known as portal hypertension, causes the veins that drain the upper portion of the stomach and the lower half of the esophagus to become tortuous and dilated like the varicose veins some people develop in their legs. Children with portal hypertension live under a Sword of Damocles, subject at any moment to life-threatening hemorrhage from rupture of one of these esophageal varices.

Many attempts were made to lower the portal pressure, but when these failed there seemed to be no alternative to removing the dilated veins themselves. This required removing the lower half of the esophagus, a procedure that had little appeal until a reliable operation to create a substitute esophagus was developed. There were a number of children, known all too well to the staff of the Boston Children's Hospital, for whom everything short of esophageal replacement had been attempted without success. One by one they had been sent home to survive as long as they could before, without pain or any other warning, a sudden massive hemorrhage carried them away.

Dr. Gross was very skeptical about the use of colon interposition in these children. He didn't know why, but he had a hunch that long-lasting benefit would not reward the effort. Most of Dr. Gross' hunches were right. Still, Lester Martin and Bob Allen pressed on him the argument that the operation might be better than helpless inactivity, and he allowed them to give the procedure a trial. Lester operated on a few of the children before his chief residency came to an end, but there were several left over for Bob.

The operations were essentially identical to the one Lucy had, but much more difficult because of the congested veins. The immediate results seemed satisfactory enough, but within five years all of the children bled again, and then there was nothing that could be done for them. It was bitterly disappointing, but most of the parents seemed genuinely grateful for the extra years the operation had given their children.

15

A Long Shot

My year at Boston Children's Hospital was nearly over. I had spent much of it as a spectator, watching or helping others do things I wanted to do myself. This had not bothered me much during the early months, but now I was impatient whenever I was assigned the role of assistant. Everyone in my class who had gone into pediatrics was either in practice or completing his last year of training. I wasn't even halfway through. Still, it never occurred to me to wonder whether or not I had been wise to switch from pediatrics to surgery. I couldn't imagine being anything but a children's surgeon.

In many ways this had been the most memorable of my training years. One of my few regrets was that my good friend and next-door neighbor Hardy Hendren had been away at the Massachusetts General Hospital for the entire year. He had greatly influenced my decision to become a surgeon, and we had looked forward to working together under Dr. Gross, but Hardy did not return to Children's until after I had gone back to City Hospital. Thereafter, he finished his training under Dr. Gross and worked briefly as a staff surgeon at Children's before establishing the pediatric surgical service at Massachusetts General, which he has headed ever since.

Hardy knew that a surgeon extends his influence by becoming a great teacher. He was a natural public speaker and knew the value of having good photographic slides with which to illustrate his talks. He bought an Exacta, a single lens reflex camera, and took hundreds of pictures in the clinics, on the wards, and in the operating rooms. He soon convinced me that I would never make the big leagues in pediatric surgery if I failed to photograph the remarkable collection of patients I saw every day. I bought a camera just like Hardy's.

When my first roll of film was developed I hurried down to the corner drug store to collect it. There were some good views of children with various disorders and some overexposed pictures of the front entrance to the hospital. The last picture was a close-up of an infant's face. There was no deformity that I could see, no birthmark or other abnormality. For the life of me I couldn't remember why I had taken that picture. I wondered about it all the way home. It was only when I projected it on a screen that I recognized my son Peter. I was receiving a priceless surgical education, but the long hours in the hospital were making me a stranger to my family.

Shortly before my year ended I made an appointment to discuss my future with Dr. Gross. According to my calculations I would finish my chief residency in general surgery in June of 1960, some two and a half years hence, and then would be ready to return for the senior residency at Boston Children's. I had worked very hard, and I thought I had done a good job. I felt I had earned a chance to come back, but it wasn't as simple as that. There was only one opening in the summer of 1960, and Dr. Gross had a long list of applicants whose chiefs were backing them as vigorously as Dr. Child could be expected to back me. There was one thing some of these candidates had that I did not. They were being sponsored by chiefs who wanted to establish new departments of pediatric surgery. When all else was equal, Dr. Gross could be expected to give the appointment to the candidate who had the most important job waiting for him. Here Dr. Child was powerless to help me. There already was a department of pediatric surgery at Boston City Hospital. Dr. Child did not need even a junior staff surgeon, let alone a department head.

Dr. Gross scanned his list of applicants and hunched his shoulders. That was a very bad sign.

"Tom," he said, "I'd put you a lot closer to the top of the list now than I would have when you came here, but I don't think you'll get the job." Had I been willing to accept this verdict, he might have gone on to give me all sorts of helpful advice as to alternative ways to achieve my goal, but it never occurred to me to ask him for it. I was absolutely convinced that I could surmount all obstacles. After all, he hadn't said "No." He had said "I don't think . . ."

"Well, sir," I said, "thank you for everything you did for me this year. Keep me on the list, because I really do want to come back." He hunched his shoulders again and put the list back in the drawer. I would have given anything to know who else was on it.

During the last few months I had grown very fond of Bob Allen. He was an excellent surgeon, a good teacher, and exceedingly generous. The events surrounding his departure from Boston Children's Hospital took place after I left, but they bear recounting.

A search committee from the children's hospital in Memphis came to Boston hoping to lure away one of Dr. Gross' senior staff surgeons. Dr. Gross had known they were coming, and he had a different candidate in mind. He was satisfied that he had solved the problems that plagued his first operations with the "pump," and had brought it back from the laboratory to the operating room. He suggested that the visitors might like to watch some open heart surgery. They almost declined because they thought the operation would take all day, but the thought of attracting a staff surgeon who was familiar with this latest advance was irresistible. Surely his most trusted staff surgeon would assist Dr. Gross on so complicated a case. They agreed to stay on for an extra day.

At eight o'clock the next morning the Memphis contingent filed into the gallery overlooking Dr. Gross' operating room. Dr. Gross was nowhere in sight, nor was any other staff surgeon. Assisted by a senior and a junior resident, Bob put a little girl on the "pump," repaired the defect within her heart, and closed her chest. Then without pausing to reload the "pump," they repeated the operation on a second little girl who had the same blood type. Dr. Gross spent the morning working quietly in his office.

That afternoon, while still a resident in training, Bob Allen was appointed Chairman of a Pediatric Surgical Department.

16

Back to City Hospital

Returning from the sparkle and abundance of Children's to the dank and dingy City Hospital was like having my coach turn into a pumpkin. I kept reminding myself that the remaining two and a half years would soon be over, but they loomed ahead of me like an eternity. Fortunately, I was soon too busy to feel sorry for myself.

I was assigned to the emergency room, where an intern took care of the cuts and bruises while a senior medical resident and I sorted out the sick people. It was not essential that we figure out exactly what was wrong with them. We merely had to start them off in the right direction, making sure that those who should be admitted to the hospital were not sent home, and that those who needed operations were not sequestered on a medical ward. Sometimes implementing the proper decision took more tact than skill, but on the whole the cooperation between the services was remarkably good. Whenever we reached an impasse the chief residents came down and took the decision out of our hands.

One of the common problems we had to settle was what to do with unconscious people. Many of them had strokes and were admitted to the medical service as soon as the diagnosis was established. A few had diabetic coma, which was easy to diagnose. They also went promptly to a medical ward. Drug abuse was not very common, but alcohol was as abundant as it is today. The medical service took care of the drunks, provided intoxication was their only problem. There was more than an occasional patient whose breath reeked of cheap wine but whose real problem was an intracranial hemorrhage caused by a rock or a short length of pipe. There were lots of barroom brawls in Boston.

To my surprise the neurosurgeons did not take care of all of the patients with head injuries. To do so would overload their service with dozens of people who merely needed a bed in which to recover without any specific treatment. The chronically overworked neurosurgeons took only the few who needed immediate brain surgery. The general surgeons took the rest. This did not make sense medically, but it was a fact of life. Drs. Ingraham and Matson had taught me to recognize the indications for emergency neurosurgical operations, and to the best of my knowledge I did not make any serious mistakes in sorting out the dozens of head-injured patients I saw in the emergency room.

Among our frequent visitors was a man of undetermined age or address named Clancy. Scarcely a Saturday night went by without an ambulance delivering Clancy to our door. His balding scalp was covered with scars resulting from wounds inflicted over the years by his drinking companions. He usually had a fresh cut or two for the intern to suture. We hated to see him come so often, but he really wasn't much trouble. He was always too comatose to move.

Skull x-rays are of less value than is generally believed, but they were ordered routinely for every unconscious patient. I often felt their chief value was that the time required to take them gave the doctor a chance to think. Clancy had a thick folder of skull x-rays, and many an intern learned from him the value of comparing the new x-ray, still wet from the developer, with those taken on previous occasions. Harried neurosurgeons, roused from precious sleep to look at x-rays showing the bullet in Clancy's head, were merciless in pointing out that it had been there for years and obviously was not responsible for his present problem.

The fact that the Harvard, Tufts, and Boston University services each ran the emergency room for eight hours a day was a godsend because, although I worked there for two solid months without a day off, I worked only eight hours a day and was able to become reacquainted with my family and keep up with my sleep. The arrangement also made it easier to find out what happened to patients after they were admitted to the hospital, since all those admitted on my shift went to the Tufts service where I could find them without having to search all over the hospital. These follow-up visits were especially helpful to me because while I had been away I had missed some valuable rotations. Keeping track of the patients I sent off to thoracic surgery, gynecology, and urology gave me a chance to learn a great deal about these disciplines, knowledge without which no surgeon's education is complete. I doubt that I could pass the general surgery exam today on the basis of what I learned in this informal and haphazard way, but it was far better than nothing, and when I later took the exam I did pass it.

Dr. Child saw to it that I did not miss the rotation on the Shortell fracture unit. Fractures at Boston City Hospital were treated in a unit that contrasted sharply with the other parts of the emergency room. It was named for a Dr. Shortell who had been dead for some years. Where the money to build this unit came from I have no idea, nor have I ever heard how the funds to support it were protected from being siphoned off to meet other needs. Whatever the explanation, the Shortell unit was as clean, bright, spacious, and well-equipped as any unit in the most luxurious of Boston's hospitals. It was always filled with patients, and within a few weeks one could see almost every variation of the common fractures. The x-ray equipment was the most modern available and the technicians so thoroughly trained that the x-rays were invariably of superb quality. The orthopedic residents handled the complicated fractures, but there were plenty of patients for all of us. We were assisted by three orderlies with special orthopedic training. They loved their work, and the casts they put on were works of art. Because we all wore the same scrub suits to keep from getting plaster on our clothes, the orderlies were frequently mistaken for doctors. They knew more about fractures than most doctors would ever learn. By their standards the first casts I put on were crude indeed, but they soon showed me how to improve, and by the time I left I thought that at least a few of my casts were works of art too.

The Shortell unit was organized to make it easy to follow patients as their fractures healed. They all returned regularly to the unit, broken ankles on Mondays, broken arms on Thursdays, and so on. The staff orthopedists who supervised these follow-up sessions had seen huge numbers of fractures and were wonderful teachers. The most devoted of them was Dr. Alexander Aitken, who like myself, had a special interest in children.

Children's bones heal quickly, often nearly twice as fast as those of adults. It is not always necessary that the ends of the broken bones be perfectly repositioned; if they touch each other at all they will often heal solidly. If the ends overlap they will heal side to side as firmly as they would had they been held end on end, but the bone will be shorter than normal. Nature corrects this shortening to some extent, but nature has its limits. If the broken pieces of bone heal at an angle there is little nature can do about the resulting deformity. Therefore, it is most important when setting children's fractures to avoid significant angulation and excessive shortening. Given half a chance children generally do very well indeed.

There is one group of fractures in children that do not give uniformly good results. This is the group in which the fracture crosses the epiphysis. The long bones of the arms and legs, and some other bones as well, have growth centers near their ends from which they derive most of their length. The portion beyond the growth center, nearest the joint, is called the epiphysis. When the epiphysis is broken off from the shaft of the bone, the growth center comes off with it. If it is accurately replaced, it usually continues to grow normally unless it has been severely crushed. If the fracture is allowed to heal at an angle, the deformity becomes progressively worse as growth continues. The most difficult of these fractures are the ones in which the fracture line goes through the growth center at an angle, dividing it into two or more pieces. These may subsequently grow at different rates, producing a deformity that becomes gradually and progressively worse until the bone stops growing at maturity. The slowly growing portions cannot be made to speed up, but the faster ones can be made to slow down by placing metal staples across them. When this is necessary, the earlier this is done, the better the final result.

Because bone grows so slowly and children's fractures heal so quickly many children have been dismissed from follow-up before the disordered growth has become apparent. Dr. Aitken followed every child with an epiphyseal injury until all growth had stopped. Since this does not happen until the late teens, many of the children in his clinics had fractures they sustained ten or more years earlier. It was a remarkable experience to see so many children who had been diligently followed for so long.

Dr. Aitken had published many articles on epiphyseal injuries. His classification of the various types was used by orthopedists around the world to identify children who required especially careful follow-up in order to detect abnormal growth at the earliest possible moment. It seems odd, perhaps, that treatment consists in using staples to arrest the growth of the part of the bone that is growing normally, but a slightly short arm or leg that is straight is vastly preferable to one of normal length that has been allowed to grow crooked.

A number of small children came to the Shortell unit with a simple problem known as "nursemaid's elbow," a name presumably retained from a more affluent era. Very few of the children we saw at the City Hospital had nursemaids.

The story was always the same. The child had suddenly stopped using his arm, which hung limply from his shoulder. It appeared to cause little or no pain as long as he did not try to do anything with it. There was no swelling or tenderness. Because the whole arm appeared to be involved the unwary often suspected that the trouble was in the shoulder, but although the child would not move it himself, he would allow the doctor to put his shoulder through a full range of motion without protest.

If x-rays were taken the bones in the affected arm appeared identical to those in the normal arm. This was because the trouble was near the elbow joint, and in little children the ends of the bones that make up the joints have so little calcium in them that they are invisible on x-rays.

The child's problem was easily and painlessly cured by flexing his elbow at a right angle with his forearm in front of his chest and turning his hand so that the palm faced forward. There were other equally effective maneuvers. Everyone had his favorite. With a hand over the lateral side of the elbow the doctor could feel a distinct click as the round head of the radius slipped back to its normal position within the circular fibers of the annular ligament from which it had been partially dislocated by a pull on the child's outstretched arm.

When questioned about this pull the parents always gave some version of the same story. The child had been snatched from danger. He had accidentally stepped down from a curb, a distance in his terms equal to that of an adult stepping down from a dining room table. The parent was playfully swinging the child around by the arm. The variations were endless but the theme was the same—a sudden pull on the outstretched arm. "It wasn't the arm," the saying went, "it was the jerk on the end." Many parents sheepishly agreed.

Throughout our training we were encouraged to write articles for publication in medical journals. The meticulous records in the Shortell unit were a gold mine of clinical material, and I decided to look up and report the hospital's experience with osteomyelitis in children. I was able to summarize the progress of a large series of infants and children with infections of the bones and joints. These ranged from inconsequential to devastating, depending on which bones were affected, what the offending bacterium was, and how rapidly they were recognized and treated. There were a few children with tuberculosis, and they usually ended up with terrible results, but the most recent of them had been treated with the new antituberculous drugs and fared much better. Many of the infants were infected with pneumococci. If treated promptly they all did well because all pneumococci were very sensitive to penicillin. Most of the other children were infected with staphylococci.

When it was first introduced, shortly after Pearl Harbor, penicillin killed nearly all staphylococci, but in the ensuing years strain after strain became resistant to it. The children whose staphylococci were sensitive to penicillin responded much more favorably to it than those who required treatment with the newer "wonder drugs," even though in the laboratory these drugs seemed equally effective. Dr. Maxwell Finland, who was a world authority in the field of antibiotic therapy, worked at the City Hospital, and everyone depended on him to select the antibiotic most suitable for each patient. He advised that every child with osteomyelitis be started on penicillin while he tested their bacteria against all the available drugs, a process that sometimes took as long as a week. His explanation as to why penicillin worked better than the other antibiotics was that it penetrated the bone better. He was a wise clinician and he was probably right. My article, summarizing seventy-three cases of infections of the bones and joints in children was accepted for publication in the *New England Journal of Medicine* where it finally appeared in April of 1960, three months before I left the City Hospital. It is obsolete now, but at the time I was very proud of it.

17

Two Teachers

The children's building at the City Hospital had been built in 1933 while James Michael Curley was mayor of Boston. It did not boast a lobby, but it had a small vestibule dominated by a large portrait of Mrs. Curley, who had been, according to a little brass plaque, "An Exemplary Boston Mother." If it was a true likeness, Mrs. Curley had at least been lovely to look at.

The people of Boston adored Mr. Curley despite some pretty convincing evidence that he was a crook. They had even gone so far as to re-elect him to office while he was serving time in jail. It was said that his lawyer had won his freedom by convincing a judge that Mr. Curley was suffering simultaneously from eight fatal diseases. He was now an old man, no longer active in the political affairs he had dominated for forty years, but the people's affection for him was as strong as ever. He was a tough old bird, but he did need hospitalization from time to time, and he always came to Boston City Hospital. During one of these admissions a colleague of mine was assigned to help take care of him. Looking out of the old man's window at the children's building across the parking lot, my friend expressed admiration that Mr. Curley had generously given the poor sick children of Boston so fine a structure. Mr. Curley replied with a twinkle in his eye that he had stolen from the citizens of Boston three times what the building had cost.

The hospital had a good Pediatric Department headed by Dr.

Sidney Gellis, who had helped me by suggesting that I send Dr. Gross a telegram. Dr. Gellis was new at his job at the City Hospital, but he was beginning to attract a few of the best graduating medical students to his internship and residency program. He faced stiff competition because in addition to Boston Children's, the Massachusetts General Hospital had a strong Pediatric Department with a galaxy of Harvard professors, and Tufts University had the venerable Floating Hospital.

This hospital no longer floats, but it actually did derive from a hospital ship that took infants out on the salt water to escape the pestilent vapors of the city. This was thought to offer them the best hope of surviving the scourge of infant diarrhea which killed hundreds of babies every year. After it was learned that salt water was more effective when given by vein, the ship was abandoned, but the name persists.

As yet, the Massachusetts General Hospital had no pediatric surgeon, but the Floating Hospital had a very good one in Dr. Orvar Swensen. His service was somewhat smaller than the one at Boston Children's, but it was very highly regarded, and together they dwarfed the pediatric surgical service at Boston City Hospital when I began my six-month tour as its chief resident in January 1959.

My department chief was Dr. John Chamberlain. His was a part-time job for which he received the title of Clinical Professor but no pay. Like Drs. Crandon and Flynn, he had made Boston City Hospital a part of his very being and never stopped to question why he was so devoted to it. He had none of Dr. Gross' driving ambition and none of Dr. Child's preoccupation with minutiae. Nor did he suffer, as they did, from an almost desperate need to remain aloof. He was compassionate, gregarious, and as open as all outdoors. He lived by Alexander Pope's advice: "Be not the first by whom the new is tried,/Nor yet the last to lay the old aside." He performed conventional, uncomplicated operations from which his patients made serene, uncomplicated recoveries.

Most of his patients came to him from the health service of the Massachusetts Institute of Technology. The students usually presented problems related to appendicitis, injuries, or gynecology. The faculty had more than their share of ulcers, which were treated surgically more often than they are now, as well as the usual variety of middle-age complaints. Many of them prevailed upon Dr. Chamberlain to operate on their parents, aunts, uncles, and grandparents. His practice ranged from infancy to extreme old age, and he brought to pediatric surgery a broader perspective than specialists like Dr. Gross and Dr. Swensen.

On New Year's Day Dr. Chamberlain and I made rounds together for the first time. He was delighted to have a resident with some pediatric experience, and I knew at once that working for him was going to be a pleasure. Most of the children on the surgical service were in the hospital because they had been injured. As we came to the bed of a perky red-headed boy who had been thrown from a moving automobile Dr. Chamberlain pointed out how easy it would have been to prevent this from happening. "Doctors don't do enough about preventing accidents," he said. It was obviously true, but he was the first surgeon I had ever met who appeared to have given any thought to the idea.

The next little boy we came to had run into the street and been hit by a car. Quick thinking and bold action by Chris Economopoulis, who had preceded me as Dr. Chamberlain's resident, had saved the boy's life. Apparently Chris had lived up to his old refrain, "I have to learn." Dr. Chamberlain remarked that the best way to tell if a surgeon was really good was to watch how he cared for an injured child. In the next six months he would guide me in caring for more than a hundred injured children, and the lessons he taught me would form the cornerstone of my surgical career.

My first injured child arrived just as we were finishing our rounds, and Dr. Chamberlain came down with me to the emergency room to see him. He was a twelve-year-old boy who had slid off a toboggan into a tree. He was pale and thirsty and grunted every time he took a breath. He complained bitterly of pain in his abdomen, which was very tender and appeared slightly distended. I examined him and told Dr. Chamberlain I felt we should operate on him, but I hadn't the slightest idea what we would find in his abdomen. I drew a blood sample for the blood bank to cross-match and filled out some x-ray requisitions.

"How much blood did you order?" Dr. Chamberlain asked casually. I had ordered one pint. "Better make that six," he said. The x-rays I had ordered were canceled and the boy was in the operating room at least an hour earlier than he would have been had I been left to my own devices. His abdomen had increased considerably in girth in the few moments since he had left the emergency room. It contained at least three pints of blood which we had to siphon away before we could see that more was pouring from a huge laceration in the liver. Dr. Chamberlain calmly compressed the liver with his hands and the bleeding stopped, but it started up again every time he relaxed his grip. By the time I had repaired the laceration and stopped the bleeding the last of the six pints of blood was running into a vein in the boy's arm as fast as the anesthetist could pump it.

Speed is the essence of good trauma care. If Dr. Chamberlain had not been there I would have been five pints short and almost an hour too late. I would have known the unimportant fact that the boy had three broken ribs, because I would have delayed the operation to obtain unnecessary x-rays, but the fractures would have been found in the autopsy room anyway. As it was, the boy went home about a week after his operation, bitterly disappointed because we wouldn't let him play hockey until the next winter.

Sharing Dr. Chamberlain's part-time duties, in the role of Assistant Chief of Pediatric Surgery, was Dr. Kenneth Welch. He was younger and more recently trained than Dr. Chamberlain, and he confined his practice exclusively to children. He had a special interest in cleft lips and cleft palates, which he repaired with more skill and refined technique than any other surgeon I have ever seen. He was a world authority on pectus excavatum, or funnel chest. Because of Dr. Welch I saw many more children with this condition at the City Hospital than I had at Children's.

Funnel chest is primarily of cosmetic importance. It is rarely treated in girls, because when they are young they appear unaware that they have a depression in the middle of their chests, and it actually enhances their appearance when they mature. Boys with similar deformities often develop severe psychological problems as they enter the teens. Although the depression can only be cured by creating a large scar, nearly all boys with the malformation are eager to have it corrected.

The upper seven or eight ribs on each side of the chest are joined to the sternum, or breastbone, by strips of cartilage. The cause of funnel chest is not completely understood, but is thought to be a derangement in the growth of these little strips of cartilage causing them to force the lower portion of the sternum inward. As the sternum presses on the front of the heart it often displaces it, giving the child's chest x-ray an unusual appearance and causing standard electrocardiograms to appear abnormal. If allowances are made for the displaced position of the heart, the electrocardiogram is normal, and cardiac function is rarely if ever affected. Expansion of the lungs may be slightly compromised, but usually this is compensated for by lateral growth of the ribs, so that although the chest is shallow it is wider than normal.

Dr. Welch had done some studies that seemed to show that breathing improved after the operation. He firmly believed that boys could run faster and swim farther, but the scientific validity of his studies was questioned by a number of his critics. Usually six months to a year separated the pre- and postoperative studies. During this time the children had grown significantly and may have become less fearful of the testing apparatus, both of which would result in better scores. A serious drawback was the paucity of normal children studied at similar intervals. Dr. Welch did not emphasize the possibility of respiratory improvement as much as his critics thought he did, and he carefully pointed out to parents, at least when I was with him, that the primary benefits of the operation were cosmetic and psychological. Of these benefits there were no doubters.

Dr. Welch helped me do a number of operations on boys with pectus excavatum. The objective was to bring the lower portion of the sternum forward and remove the deformed cartilages in such a way that new cartilages could grow to meet the sternum in its corrected position. To do this we made incisions in the perichondrium, the delicate sheath of tissue that surrounds and nourishes the cartilage. Using instruments, some of which were dental tools given Dr. Welch by an oral surgeon, we gently stripped off the sleeve of tenacious but easily torn perichondrium and carefully removed the cartilage from inside it. The collar bones and the upper two cartilages on each side are attached to the manubrium, the square plate of bone with a prominent notch at the top that comprises the upper portion of the sternum. These upper cartilages are usually not deformed and are left intact. At the bottom of the manubrium the sternum takes a rather sharp bend inward in boys with pectus excavatum. Although the depression appears to curve as seen beneath the skin, the sternum below this angulation is actually almost straight. A single wedge-shaped cut through the front of the bone allows the sternum to be brought forward, carrying with it the inner ends of the empty perichondrial sheaths.

Three or four large sutures placed across this transverse defect and tied securely hold the lower piece of the sternum in its new forward position. Dr. Welch did not use any other form of immobilization, though some other surgeons make a hoop of wire with foam-rubber padding on the ends which they fix to the skin with adhesive tape. To this hoop they tie a large suture from the lower end of the sternum as added protection against a cave-in during the two or three weeks it takes the bone to heal. Dr. Welch felt this hoop was unnecessary, and I never had occasion later to wish I had used one.

The little slits in the perichondrial sheaths are carefully repaired with fine sutures. Within a month or six weeks they fill completely with new cartilage. The muscles of the chest wall that were retracted out of the way are replaced in their normal position and the long skin incision carefully closed. If the operation is done properly, only two or three ounces of blood are lost and blood transfusion is not needed. Dr. Welch prided himself in being able to remove four to six cartilages from each side of the chest without puncturing the back of any of the perichondrial sheaths. If this occurred, air entered the chest and the lung collapsed; an event that wounded his pride but was of little consequence if the anesthetist inflated the lung completely and drove the air out again while we closed the little tear.

One problem with repair of pectus excavatum is that a generous incision is needed, and despite our best efforts to close the skin carefully the scar was much more unsightly than a scar of similar size would have been on the abdomen or in the groin. Perhaps this is because on the front of the chest there is so little fat beneath the skin. An unsightly scar is a small price to pay for a life-saving operation on the heart or lungs, but it can be distressing when the primary objective is cosmetic. Dr. Welch found that a transverse scar running from just below one nipple to just below the other was preferable to a vertical one, but he was always disappointed that he could not produce the same nearly invisible scar that is easy to make in the groin. Ironically, these hairline scars in the groin are almost always covered by clothing whereas the front of the chest is not. Nobody else has been able to solve the scar-on-the-chest problem either, but boys who have been relieved of the hated depression in the center of their chests never seem to care.

18

Burns

In addition to many children injured by automobiles, falls, and athletic mishaps, we admitted an average of four burned children to our service every week. At least an equal number, less severely burned, were treated in the emergency room and sent home to be followed in the pediatric surgical clinic. Since I was in charge of these clinic patients as well as those in the hospital, I was responsible for more than two hundred burned children during the six months I worked with Drs. Chamberlain and Welch.

The two men were very different in age, training, and temperament, but they worked very well together. The plan they formulated for the care of burned children was clearer, more specific, and more easily understood than any I could find in the medical literature. Some changes have since been made, but for the most part the principles they taught me are still valid.

The arrival in the emergency room of a seriously burned child can be an unnerving experience. The child is invariably in pain and often very frightened. The anxiety of the parents is augmented, sometimes enormously, by guilt. Whether they acknowledge it or not, they always believe that had they not somehow failed in their role as parents the terrible accident would not have occurred. Most are openly fearful or downright hysterical. It is relatively easy to help them. A few appear indifferent or inappropriately nonchalant. Their true feelings are deeply repressed, and they are the ones who will have the most difficulty in coming to terms with reality in the days ahead. Dealing effectively with burned children and their parents can challenge the most seasoned clinician.

Getting off to the right start depends on being able to answer several crucial questions. Does the child need to be admitted to the hospital? Will he develop breathing difficulty? Will he need to be given intravenous fluids? Will he need skin grafts? Will he live? How long will he have to stay in the hospital? What will he look like when he goes home? It is usually possible to answer all of these questions with great accuracy while the child is still in the emergency room, and nothing is more reassuring to confused and anxious parents than giving them the answers openly, honestly, and promptly without having to be asked.

There are basically three reasons to admit children with burns to a hospital. A few develop severe breathing difficulties several hours after being burned. When first seen they may appear entirely normal, but often the telltale signs of impending trouble can be found. These include a change of voice, which at first may be so subtle that only those familiar with the child can recognize it, but which progresses to obvious hoarseness in a few hours. Scalding water virtually never causes breathing difficulty, and flame in the presence of an abundance of oxygen is not likely to. Thus, scalded children and those whose snowsuits catch fire in a pile of burning leaves are unlikely to have respiratory trouble. It is children burned inside buildings where the supply of air is limited who are candidates for trouble. If respiratory embarrassment is the only concern, hospitalization for forty-eight hours is sufficient to prevent an occasional disaster.

The second reason for hospitalization is to provide intravenous fluids. Burned tissue swells in a very predictable way as water leaks out of the injured capillaries. Nothing can be done to prevent this, but the leakage causes no problem if the fluid that is lost into the tissues is replaced at the appropriate rate. The rules that govern fluid administration in adults cannot be scaled down for children without important modifications. Children normally require fluid at a much more rapid rate than adults. A mother who takes her newborn baby home from the hospital soon finds that he cannot sleep through the night without being fed. It isn't the calories he needs so desperately; it is the fluid. At seven pounds he consumes three ounces of fluid every four hours around the clock. If his mother, at a hundred and twenty pounds, continued to take in fluid at the same rate she would have to drink two and a half quarts with each meal and two and a half more at bed time. Small wonder that children need vigorous intravenous support when a burn is superimposed on their normal fluid needs!

The severity of a burn depends on both its depth and its extent. The depth has great bearing on its ability to heal but surprisingly little effect on the amount of fluid leaked by the injured capillaries. Therefore, the amount of fluid that must be given a burned child depends mainly on the extent of the wound; i.e., the percent of his total body surface that has been burned. Here again, children are different. Compared to the rest of the body, an infant's head is twice as big as that of an adult, whereas his legs are proportionately smaller. Little children frequently scald themselves by pulling hot water down on their heads as they reach up to the inviting handle of a pot on a stove or trip over the cord of an electric percolator. The resulting burn on the head affects nearly twice as large a fraction of a two-year-old child's skin as it would were he an adult. Conversely, if he scalds his legs by becoming trapped in a tub of hot water, the burn is less extensive than a similar burn in an adult because an adult has a considerably greater percentage of his skin on his legs.

These differences between small children and adults are not difficult to understand, but serious miscalculations are bound to occur if they are ignored. Dr. Chamberlain's rule called for admitting to the hospital all preschool children with burns of over 10 percent of their skin, whereas teenagers could safely go home unless more than 20 percent of their skin was burned. The primary reason for admitting little children to the hospital was to ensure that they received the fluids they needed intravenously. Experience has shown over and over again that beyond these limits children cannot be depended on to satisfy their tremendous needs by drinking, no matter how attentively they are cared for.

The third major problem involves healing the wound. Here the depth of injury is the primary concern. The wound can heal of its own accord if the deepest layer of the skin survives, since it is from this deepest layer that new skin is generated. But the damage caused by the burn itself is only part of the problem. While the germinative layer has wonderful powers to regenerate, it is far less resistant to infection than are the outer layers. When these protective layers are destroyed an uncontrolled multiplication of bacteria can easily kill the delicate germinative layer, leading to the formation of ugly scars and often making skin grafting necessary. The essence of burn-wound care is preventing infection, using methods that are acceptably free from pain.

In the hospital it was possible to treat children with superficial burns simply by exposing them to the air. They were placed in cribs with sterilized sheets that were changed frequently. At first the wounds were red and moist, but after a day or two a thin brownish crust appeared on the surface. As soon as this became firm and dry the children could be allowed to run about the ward and could eat their meals with their playmates at a little table near the kitchen.

After ten to fourteen days the crust would fall off and the skin beneath it would be intact. At first it was pinker than normal, and in black children devoid of pigment, but within a year all traces of the burn would vanish. The crust was not the least bit painful, but it did require attentive care by the nurses to keep it clean and dry. An occasional mother could accomplish this at home, but most could not. Even in the 1950s a surprising number of mothers worked outside the home, and others with several small children to look after simply did not have the confidence or the time to do it well. We admitted many children with small wounds to the hospital who could have cared for themselves at home had they been adults.

An alternative might have been to provide a sterile dressing for the wound, but bulky bandages and the primitive antibacterial ointments then available did not prevent infection as reliably as exposure to the air. Bandages could prevent new bacteria from being smeared on the wounds, but many bacteria were already there from the moment of burning. No method of actually sterilizing the skin has ever been found, and even today the goal must be to discourage bacteria from multiplying. Eliminating them is the utopia we all long for but have never seen.

About two thirds of all burned children are scalded by hot liquid. Usually this is some form of water, either cooking or bath water, coffee, tea, soup, or cereal. Occasionally it is boiling when it comes in contact with the skin, but often it is somewhat cooler. Scalding injuries tend to spare the deepest layer of the skin and permit spontaneous healing. Full-thickness burns can be produced if boiling water is held in contact with the skin by heavy clothing, but this is the exception rather than the rule. Grease, on the other hand, can be heated much hotter than water, and grease burns are often much deeper than water burns. Whenever flame is involved, especially when clothing catches fire, a deep burn is nearly always produced.

Cathy was typical of a number of children burned by flame. She was wearing a pretty blue party dress made of a highly flammable synthetic material which she set on fire in an all too common way, by playing with matches. The fabric shrank as it burned, clinging tenaciously to her body, charring the skin and even burning the fat beneath it. Her mother smothered the flames with a blanket, undoubtedly saving Cathy's life, and brought her quickly to the hospital. The front of her body was burned from the tip of her chin to below her navel, but fortunately her face, arms and legs were spared.

After a few days her wound was covered with a thick leathery eschar. We knew that beneath it there was no viable skin, and that she would require extensive skin grafting when the eschar separated away. To hasten this separation we used an enzyme made from the bark of fig trees and marketed under the name of Debricin. This produced some pain, but the pain lasted for only about twenty minutes, and Cathy bravely put up with it when we applied the Debricin every eight hours. The objective was to remove the eschar quickly so that we could apply skin grafts before the bacteria had a chance to multiply to dangerous numbers.

Cathy's mother wanted desperately to donate skin to cover her daughter's wound. To have allowed her to do so would have been profoundly beneficial, for it would have relieved her guilt by allowing her to repay Cathy for failing to keep the matches out of reach. Had Cathy's wound been more extensive we might have considered using some of her mother's skin. Eventually it would have been rejected, but as a temporary cover it could have been valuable. As it was, Cathy's entire wound could be covered with her own skin at one operation, so we declined her mother's offer.

By the twelfth day the Debricin had caused all of the eschar to separate from Cathy's wound. There was no sign of infection. We took her to the operating room, and using an electric dermatome, which resembled a large electric hair clipper, we removed strips of skin from Cathy's thighs. The dermatome had a little knob which controlled the thickness of the skin grafts, and it was set so that only the outer layer of the skin was removed. The areas from which the grafts were taken would heal in about two weeks, leaving only faint marks. The strips of skin, resembling very thin strips of bacon, were laid on the wound, covering the burned areas of her neck, chest and abdomen. A few sutures and a large dressing applied with great care held the grafts in place.

The change in Cathy was astonishing. As soon as she awoke from the anesthetic she began to demand food, which she had apathetically rejected while her wound was open. Her temperature fell to normal and remained there, in contrast to the wildly swinging fever she had had before her operation. Perhaps the biggest change was in her disposition. She had been withdrawn, whiny, and even combative, but now she was pleasant, happy, and outgoing. She had been restored to health, and it was only in retrospect that I realized how ill she had been. She had lost twelve pounds since admission to the hospital. That was comparable to an adult losing at least twenty-five pounds in less than two weeks. Had this loss gone on for another week or ten days, as it might have without the hastening effect of the Debricin, she would have been perilously ill.

We thought Debricin represented a wonderful advance because it permitted us to reduce to the absolute minimum the interval between the burn injury and complete closure of the wound by skin grafts. This was the most important factor in Cathy's recovery. Politics played a cruel joke on surgeons who valued Debricin, because Debricin came only from the bark of fig trees, and Fidel Castro controlled all the fig trees from which it came. When relations with Cuba cooled, Debricin disappeared from the market.

At the City Hospital, as at all teaching hospitals, the educational highlight of the week is Grand Rounds. These are not great processionals, as the name implies, but formal gatherings in a large auditorium. All of the clinical departments, including medicine, surgery, pediatrics, and radiology are represented. The center of attraction is a patient who either has a knotty, unsolved problem or illustrates an important teaching point. Sometimes Grand Rounds represents the ultimate decision-making conference, at which the most seasoned physicians in every specialty pool their expertise for the patient's benefit. Sometimes it is simply a "show and tell" session, which can be of tremendous teaching value if presented with sufficient showmanship to hold everyone's attention. Whatever the format, if carefully prepared and skillfully conducted, Grand Rounds provides a most effective way for physicians to keep abreast of new developments in disciplines other than their own.

The frequency with which the various departments were required to organize these weekly sessions was governed by their size. Since ours was a very small department, we were afforded this "opportunity" only once every six months. When our turn approached I scanned our list of patients to find one suitable for presentation. Timing is crucial in finding such a patient, since illness does not respect the calendar. No matter how fascinating a patient's problem may be, presenting his case after he has recovered and gone home simply is not done.

I concluded that we had no single outstanding patient and suggested that we present and discuss a series of patients representing the whole panorama of burns in childhood. Dr. Chamberlain took to the idea, and with a gleam in his eye that I recognized only in retrospect, told me to go ahead and select the children and prepare to present them. I thought that he would then discuss and summarize the plan of burn management that he and Dr. Welch had so carefully worked out but curiously had never written down. With only an hour to go I discovered that he had no intention of doing so. The entire hour and a half was up to me.

The auditorium was filled to the rafters. In the front row sat my stern and exacting chief, Dr. Child, surrounded by the heads of the major clinical services of Tufts, Boston University, and

Harvard. There were a surprising number of visitors from other hospitals. Among the visiting house officers was Judson Randolph, Dr. Gross' senior resident, who has since become Chief of Surgery at the Children's Hospital in Washington, D.C. He currently held the position to which I hoped to be appointed when my years at the City Hospital were over. As I began my presentation I felt as if the entire medical world were watching.

I had many colored slides showing the progress of each of the children. As the first of these slides appeared on the giant screen I silently thanked Hardy Hendren for talking me into buying my trusty Exacta. Fortunately, I had a very clear idea of what I had expected Dr. Chamberlain to say after I presented the children and described their problems. The hour and a half went by without a hitch, and when it was over both Dr. Chamberlain and Dr. Welch were very pleased. Even Dr. Child gave me a nod of approval as he left.

Soon afterward Dr. Gross' secretary called to request that I repeat the presentation at Boston Children's. Jud Randolph had evidently given him a favorable account of my discussion of a problem rarely seen at Children's. For some reason, burned children seldom went there. Realizing the influence this opportunity might have on Dr. Gross' decision to offer me a senior residency, I carefully polished and endlessly rehearsed my presentation, which had to be modified to be effective without showing live patients. When it was over Dr. Gross was very complimentary but carefully avoided giving me an opportunity to reiterate my desire to return to his service. Nevertheless, I went back to the City Hospital greatly encouraged.

Dr. Welch decided we should have large transparencies made from my slides for an exhibit at the annual AMA convention in Atlantic City. As a reward for my work, and in order to have an extra person to man the exhibit, he and Dr. Chamberlain paid my expenses and took me with them.

Among the many visitors to our booth was Dr. J. Harold Walton, editor of the CIBA *Symposia*. This popular monthly publication had a wide circulation, not only because of Dr. Walton's ability to ferret out topics of interest, but also because of Dr. Frank Netter's colored drawings which were regarded as among the finest examples of medical illustration available anywhere in the world.

Dr. Walton persuaded Dr. Chamberlain to provide the text for an issue of the CIBA *Symposia* to be illustrated with some of my photographs and some of Dr. Netter's drawings. I was assigned to write the text, which summarized in print for the first time the plan for caring for burned children that I had learned so thoroughly. Dr. Walton was an exasperating editor whose picky fussiness almost drove me crazy, but I had to admit that the text he finally accepted was much clearer than any I could have produced without him. The photographs and Dr. Netter's drawings enhanced it greatly, and it became one of CIBA's most popular *Symposia*. My only regret was that Dr. Netter worked in complete isolation at his home on Long Island, and I never got the opportunity to meet him.

19

Chief Resident at Last!

After working for six months under Dr. Chamberlain's watchful eye I began my final year at Boston City Hospital. Dr. Child had kept his promise to appoint me chief resident. Along the way he had had to drop some good men because the pyramid could not accommodate them. The same had happened on the Harvard and Boston University services, but unlike me, the residents who made it to the top of the other pyramids had not known until the last minute that they would do so. The security I had felt all through my surgical training had been tremendously helpful to me, and I had worn Dr. Child's promise like an invisible vest of armor through the long days and nights. Neither Dr. Child nor I had mentioned it since he had given me his word five years earlier, and the notion that I should have asked for it in writing never once had crossed my mind.

I had expected Larry Tose to move up as my assistant, but illness forced him out of the program and Ike Mehrez joined the service in his place. I was disappointed, because Larry and I were good friends and had looked forward to spending this last year together, but Ike turned out to be the best assistant anyone could ask for. He was almost as tireless as Chris Economopoulis, but much more efficient. He enjoyed administrative detail and kept the service running like a well-oiled machine. He was as comfortable with adults as I with children, and though he was my junior he taught me more than I was able to teach him.

When we took them over, the wards were filled with patients neither Ike nor I had operated upon. The previous chief resident had gone on a well-deserved vacation before starting his practice, and all the other residents and interns who were familiar with the patients had moved to other rotations. The unsung heroines of these massive yearly upheavals were the nurses, to whom many a patient unknowingly owes his life. Without them we would have been utterly lost. With their help we got off to a busy but uneventful start.

Someone has likened getting through the first week in July in a teaching hospital to wading through a herd of baby ducks. Everything seems to take three times as long as it should. The new interns, who soon will be handling many details without supervision, still have to be shown how to do simple tasks like filling out x-ray requisitions. To make matters worse, in many emergency rooms the Fourth of July is the busiest day of the year. Boston City Hospital was no exception.

Ike was everywhere, countersigning interns' orders on the wards, seeing to it that lab studies were ordered on the proper forms, and helping to sort out patients in the emergency room. When two badly injured people arrived about ten minutes apart, I took one of them to the operating room and Ike took the other. By midnight, when things had finally begun to calm down, I had completely forgotten that like the interns, Ike had come to Boston City Hospital only four days before.

It was to be an eventful year. Mayor Curley, whose eight fatal diseases were finally catching up with him, fell in his home and broke his arm. Two weeks earlier he had broken his other arm in a similar fall, and now he had to be hospitalized because the two fractures made it impossible for him to care for himself. Both breaks were of a type that would heal uneventfully, given time, but the stress caused him to bleed massively from a duodenal ulcer. Dr. George Miller, who had a high-pitched voice and was known as "Squeaky" Miller to distinguish him from Dr. Harold Miller, took the old gentleman to the operating room to try to stop the bleeding.

Ike and I were on the sidelines, as Mr. Curley was a Boston University patient, but we watched intently as Squeaky prepared to pull off yet another miracle for the old man. The door of the operating room was guarded by two big, burly Irish policemen. With their permission I peeked in through the little glass port- hole. There lay His Honor, covered with surgical drapes, sur- rounded by two nurses, thirteen doctors, and an archbishop. It was one o'clock in the morning.

In twenty minutes it was over. Squeaky had gone straight to his target, found and tied the bleeding vessel, and Mr. Curley was in the recovery room. It was a brilliant *tour de force*, just enough surgery and not one bit more. The papers joyfully recorded the event next morning, and for the moment Boston City Hospital was the center of national attention. But the tri- umph was short-lived because four days later Mr. Curley died of complications no surgeon could have prevented.

The next disaster affected Ike and me more directly. Dr. Child resigned to become Chief of Surgery at the University of Michi- gan. Appointments to positions at that level go through a maze of boards and committees, and the announcement was delayed for several weeks. Dr. Child did his best to conduct business as usual, but endless meetings in Michigan kept him away much of the time. With Ike's help I was able to give our patients reasona- bly competent care on the wards, and Drs. Crandon and Nabseth bent over backward to keep us out of trouble in the operating room, but my chief residency fell far short of what it might have been with a strong chief giving me his undivided attention. In addition to the demoralizing effect of losing Dr. Child we en- dured a period of uncertainty as to who our next chief would be. Without an heir apparent many departments drift for months before a suitable new chief can be found. I had visions of finishing the entire year under makeshift staffing arrangements.

Fortunately, those in power at Tufts moved full speed ahead to fill Dr. Child's vacant chair, and soon Dr. Ralph Deterling came to take charge. Trained in a later era than Dr. Child, he thought our service very old-fashioned and managed to alienate almost everyone before he had gotten his bags unpacked. Part of his problem, of course, was that our loyalty to Dr. Child and his way of doing things was dying a predictably lingering death. I instantly decided that I neither liked nor trusted Dr. Deterling, a mistake I should have been mature enough not to make. Despite his problems of getting settled in a new home and a new job, and despite the many commitments that took him away from the hospital during his early months, Dr. Deterling did his best to put the finishing touches on my surgical training and never gave me the slightest reason to justify mistrusting him. He just wasn't Dr. Child.

Late in the fall, on a cold rainy day, I went over to Dr. Gross' office for the long-awaited decision regarding further training with him. I had carefully researched his chief residents and found that nearly twice as many of them had started as senior residents in July as in January. Since I would be free to start in July, I pictured myself in three short years finishing his chief residency.

Dr. Gross hunched his shoulders, and before he said a word I knew it was not to be. The one position upon which I had pinned all my hopes had been given to someone else. Not only had I failed in my dream of becoming a pediatric surgeon, but I had put Patty and our children through four years of hardship for nothing. I put on my raincoat and hurried into the street, hoping no one could see that I was close to tears. I reached into the pocket of my raincoat for a handkerchief and pulled out, instead, a little toy American flag. I'd seen Amy playing with that little flag a few days before. I hadn't seen her put it in my pocket. I doubt she remembers anything about it, but in the darkest hour of my life that little flag seemed to say, "We love you, Daddy. Don't be discouraged. There must be another way." If there was another way, I certainly couldn't see it on that dismal afternoon.

Within a few days I had recovered sufficiently to begin casting about for alternatives. Dr. Swensen, at the Floating Hospital, had a one-year residency which from my family's point of view would be infinitely preferable to the three years I had hoped to spend at Children's. Jeff would soon be ten years old, Kate nine, Amy seven, and Peter three. I had been on duty in one hospital or another every day and every other night since Amy was six weeks old. I went to see Dr. Swensen, who had turned a number of Dr. Gross' cast-offs into superbly trained pediatric surgeons. The position he offered was second best, but second best at the Floating Hospital under Dr. Swensen was very good indeed. He accepted me without hesitation, and I went back to work with renewed faith in myself. Again, it never occurred to me to ask for it in writing.

As the weeks went by I began to feel the confidence that comes from being chief resident. I had done most of the standard major operations myself, first with a staff surgeon assisting me and then with Ike as my assistant. I knew how to suspect the usual adult surgical diseases and how to pursue and nail down the diagnoses. Dr. Deterling felt I overprepared some of my patients, unduly delaying their operations, but Ike and I continued to do things as Dr. Child had taught us to do them, and at least made very few errors of omission.

Different as they were, Dr. Child and Dr. Deterling had one thing in common. They were fiercely committed to teaching medical students. Nothing was more certain to arouse their ire than the discovery that one of the staff surgeons had failed to meet a teaching commitment. It was part of our job as residents to fill in whenever one of the staff surgeons was delayed or forgot to show up. Ike had a genius for predicting when these lapses would occur, and between us we often gave five or six lectures a week. No topic substitutions were permitted. If it was "Jaundice in the Elderly" day, jaundice in the elderly was what we lectured about. You don't really understand anything until you can explain it to a group of students. When the questions come, if a group of smart senior medical students can't stump you, you *really* understand it. These formal teaching sessions, sometimes prepared on very short notice, did wonders for our surgical knowledge, if not for that of the poor students. I never looked forward with relish to teaching medical students, but once I started a teaching session I always enjoyed it.

By sheer accident I overheard one day that Dr. Swensen had appointed his chief resident for the following year. I knew he had; he had appointed me. Much to my dismay, the name I heard was not mine. After a sleepless night I went to see him, and sure enough, he had promised the same job to two of us. I hadn't thought to ask for it in writing. Apparently it was an honest mistake for which Dr. Swensen was genuinely sorry. He asked for forty-eight hours in which to decide what to do, and at the end of that time offered a compromise that seemed very fair under the circumstances. The other fellow, who did have it in writing, would get the residency. I would be made a junior staff man. Dr. Swensen had dug up a salary of $8,000 for the first six months. When the new budget came out he was pretty sure he could promise the same or even a little more for the last half of the year. Currently, I was making $125 a month. It was a dream come true. He would make rounds with me every day and would show me how to do all the meticulous operations for which he was justly famous. I would be handsomely paid and would spend every night at home with my family, unless I was supervising an emergency operation. Perhaps, when the year was over, he would keep me on the staff of the Floating Hospital where I could develop my own pediatric surgical practice under virtually ideal conditions.

This time I knew enough to ask for it in writing, but before the necessary papers could be drawn up lightning struck again. Dr. Swensen was appointed Chief of Surgery at the Children's Memorial Hospital in Chicago. Every residency and junior staff position in Chicago was filled. I was high and dry again. It was getting late. If my career in pediatric surgery was to be salvaged I needed a miracle, and I needed it fast.

Once again, Dr. Gellis pointed the way. "Go back and ask Dr. Gross what to do," he said. I supposed it couldn't do any harm. Back I went, remembering hopefully how pleasantly surprised I had been at our first meeting when Dr. Gross had accepted my yearning to become a surgeon.

This time he never hunched his shoulders, even once. "Tom," he said, "you can spend just so long in a white suit. You've been in training long enough. Bill Clatworthy in Columbus is scream-ing for help. Go out and help him." Help him do what? I won-dered. He couldn't possibly want a partner who had seen all the big pediatric operations but never done any. Dr. Gross must be kidding. It was an unkind time to kid anybody. I looked in his eyes, and I knew he wasn't kidding. Furthermore, I knew that until I tried to do what he advised he would make no further suggestions.

But who was Bill Clatworthy?

20

A Preview of Columbus

Bill Clatworthy was a fierce champion of causes. Everyone had strong opinions about him, though few pretended to understand him. He was at once the simplest and the most complex of men —a seething bundle of opposites. He could be sympathetic and considerate, but he could also be utterly oblivious to the needs and thoughts of others. To some he was the essence of warmth and charm; to others he was hostility personified. He had a violent temper, and spewed forth a torrent of rage at the slightest provocation, but when the fury subsided, the hapless victims of his outbursts usually conceded that he had been right.

He was a relentless taskmaster, given less to praising what pleased him than to heaping scorn on shoddy work. He considered eight hours in the life of an infant equivalent to twenty-four in the life of an adult. Because infants were subject to such rapid changes he thought pediatric surgeons had to work three times as hard as those responsible for adults, not to give infants better care, just equally good care. He was almost clairvoyantly perceptive about people and what motivated them, but he had blind spots. One of these blind spots hid from him a tragic flaw that was painfully obvious to those around him. In championing his causes he often chose to fight when a battle was not called for, and, failing to engage a worthy adversary, unwittingly turned the full force of his destructive power on himself.

Bill had trained at Boston Children's during a magnificent transition, starting under Dr. William E. Ladd and finishing under Dr. Gross. Dr. Ladd was the acknowledged father of pediatric surgery in America, the first surgeon of great stature to devote his life to the care of infants and children. It was Dr. Ladd, with the backing of the Harvard Medical School, who had established the surgical service at the Children's Hospital and set the standards for the rest of the country. He had attracted Dr. Swensen and Dr. Gross to pediatric surgery and trained them both. The two were fierce rivals who had stayed on as Dr. Ladd's associates, each hoping to succeed him when it came time for him to retire. Dr. Gross won out in the end, but not by much. To prepare for a career in pediatric surgery under any of these master surgeons would have been a privilege. To come under the influence of all three of them during one's formative years was a rare opportunity. Bill Clatworthy had made the most of it.

When Dr. Gross suggested that I join him, Bill was in his tenth year as Chief of Surgery at the Columbus Children's Hospital. On the surface, Columbus, Ohio, seemed an unlikely place in which to launch a pediatric surgical service that would become known the world over, but he succeeded in doing so. In addition to his own ability and hard work, a number of factors conspired to help him.

The Second World War imposed on all communities a long moratorium during which construction of new hospitals, and even renovation of old ones, was impossible. In Columbus a forward-looking group of civic leaders took advantage of this interim to survey the needs of the community and plan for the day when building could begin again.

Columbus was the state capital, situated almost exactly in the center of Ohio. With Cleveland more than a hundred miles to the northeast, and Cincinnati about the same distance to the southwest, Columbus was the major medical center for about four million people. It had a small children's hospital, a university hospital, and a half dozen community hospitals. The population was growing rapidly, and the hospitals were bulging at the seams. All but the maternity hospital were considered fully rounded general hospitals, capable of giving all services to all people. Most of them cared for children as well as adults. Getting the trustees of all of these hospitals to cooperate in planning for the future would have taxed the wisdom of Solomon, but co-operate they did, joining in an agreement not to include the addition of any new children's beds in their plans for expansion. Some even agreed to close the ones they had. Armed with this guarantee, and backed by enthusiastic community support, the trustees of the little children's hospital formulated ambitious plans, and when the war clouds lifted they built in Columbus one of the three largest children's hospitals in the United States.

As the hospital began to attract talented new people to its staff, it was aided by the growth and development of the College of Medicine of Ohio State University. Deans of medical schools have to raise money for bricks and mortar and they have to attract good teachers to their faculty. While they usually have some skill in both these areas, they tend to be really good at only one of them. Dean Charles Doan was good at attracting people. Despite the relatively mediocre reputation that the College of Medicine enjoyed when he took it over, he soon filled two key positions on his faculty with strong and able men who understood Bill Clatworthy and supported him. One was Earl Baxter, Chairman of Pediatrics and Chief of Staff of Children's Hospital. The other was Robert M. Zollinger, Chairman of Surgery and Surgeon-in-Chief of the University Hospital. They stood behind Bill in every one of his early battles, and he owed a large measure of his success to their unwavering support.

In the beginning Bill carried the full load alone, doing all of the teaching and research and taking over from the general surgeons a greater and greater share of the patient care. His service grew rapidly as word got about that babies with surgical conditions that had invariably been fatal were beginning to survive. Within a few years there were three pediatric surgeons in Columbus.

Tom Boles, trained in general surgery by Dr. Zollinger and in pediatric surgery by Bill, returned to his native Columbus after practicing for a short while in Seattle. Like two bulls in the same pasture, Bill and Tom admired and respected each other but never became close friends. Bob Izant, who had been senior resident on Dr. Gross' service during my first year at Boston Children's, arrived in Columbus shortly after Tom. The three men worked very effectively together, and had Bob not gone home to

Cleveland to start his own department, there would have been no opening for me when my residency came to an end in the summer of 1960.

The more I learned about Columbus and the fiery surgeon to whom Dr. Gross had directed me, the less confident I became that I represented what he would be looking for. Surely there were people with more training in pediatric surgery who would jump at the chance to work with him. I met him for the first time in an elevator in Chicago where he and Mrs. Clatworthy were attending a medical meeting. He invited Patty and me to have lunch with them. After the usual pleasantries he turned to me and asked what my experience in pediatric surgery had been.

It was a dismal interview. He listed operation after operation that he had a perfect right to expect an associate to be able to perform. Time after time my answer was the same. I had seen and participated in these operations, but I had never done them myself. When the litany was over I felt completely naked. As far as I could see, the only way I could fill his need was to begin by working for him as a resident. I was perfectly willing to do this, but he had plenty of residents. He needed help at a staff level and he needed it right away. I was certain I would soon be back in Dr. Gross' office, hat in hand, to ask where else I should look. Patty was sure I would never get a respectable position anywhere.

To our surprise Bill asked when we could come to Columbus for a preliminary visit. Convinced that the sooner we put this futile exercise behind us the better, I replied that we would like to come at the earliest opportunity, preferably before Christmas. We parted with his assurance that he would soon get in touch with us. Mrs. Clatworthy had been cheerful and effervescent when our lunch began, but she looked tired when it was over.

She was more than tired. She was seriously ill. Our visit to Columbus was postponed again and again as her condition worsened, and early in the spring we got word that she had died. Bill was devastated. They had been married only a short time, and Bill had found in this second marriage all the happiness he had missed in his first. Though we had met her only once, we had seen enough to know how profound his grief must be.

When I finally saw the Columbus Children's Hospital I knew

at once that I wanted to work there. It had a striking vitality. The department heads were far younger than their counterparts in Boston. They were doing exciting things and were obviously happy in their surroundings. The new wing of the hospital was in the last phases of construction, and noise and bustle were everywhere.

Evidently Bill was serious about giving me a try, for he had set up a series of hurdles, professional and otherwise, with which to put me through my paces. The first was a conference at the hospital at which I was asked to discuss an unusual case. I made a mess of it, not knowing the significance of the key clue, that malformations of the vertebrae in the neck were sometimes associated with malformations of the esophagus. Very few people in the audience appeared to know it either, and it didn't seem to matter.

The second hurdle was more formidable. Bill announced that we were going water-skiing. I was sure to flunk this also, as I had never even seen a pair of water-skis. Realizing that I was somewhat of a novice, Bill tossed his daughter, Suzie, into the water and told me to watch her closely. In a moment this athletic ten-year-old was swooping back and forth behind the boat, first on both skis and then on only one. Bill assured me my turn would soon be coming. Suzie could have skied until sundown as far as I was concerned.

Eventually Bill hauled her into the boat and I faced my moment of truth. I gathered the skis beneath me, clutched the rope and nodded. The boat roared away, and to my amazement I was up and skiing. I had stood up on my very first try. I remained upright for about two hundred feet, and was beginning to gloat over this minor triumph when the rope abruptly slackened and I fell in a heap. The boat had hit a log floating beneath the surface of the water and wrecked the propeller. Water-skiing was over for the day. Bill was the soul of concern that I hadn't been able to show my stuff. We limped slowly back to the dock, and I never went water-skiing again, ever.

The third hurdle was Grand Rounds. At last I was in my element. The little girl whose case I was asked to discuss had a severe burn. Thanks to Dr. Chamberlain and Dr. Welch I had an answer for every question, and the hour was over before I knew it.

Bill offered me a chance to join him, contingent on the approval of Dr. Baxter and Dr. Zollinger. Fortunately, Dr. Baxter had missed my discussion of the baby with the malformed esophagus but had been in the front row when I discussed the treatment of burns. In a brief, cordial interview he told me he would welcome me to the staff. He told me how proud he was of the way the hospital was growing and of the fine group of pediatricians he was assembling. He assured me that I would find these pediatricians, upon whom I would depend for the referral of my patients, a competent and supportive group of friends. In a fatherly way he urged me to come to him without the slightest hesitation if I ever had a problem. It was easy to see why everyone loved and admired Dr. Baxter.

Dr. Zollinger's approval was important in ways I hadn't thought much about. In Boston Dr. Gross had appeared essentially autonomous. If he had been responsible to anyone but the dean of the Harvard Medical School, whose name I didn't even know, it certainly had not been obvious to me. In Ohio it was different. Bill served at the pleasure of the Chairman of the Department of Surgery, and Dr. Zollinger lost no opportunity to make this clear. I had assumed that my primary function as a pediatric surgeon would be to take care of patients, with teaching and research as secondary sidelines. Not so. Although patient care would occupy a major share of my time and would supply almost all of my income, my privilege to take care of patients in a teaching hospital was contingent on my satisfactory performance as a teacher. Research could wait a few months while I learned the ropes, but within a reasonable period I was to produce meaningful research as well. If I didn't, my appointment, which came up for renewal every year, simply wouldn't be renewed.

Dr. Zollinger was out of town, so I would have to meet him later. Patty and I flew back to Boston, elated at what had happened so far. As we boarded the plane it dawned on me that we hadn't met Tom Boles. Like Dr. Zollinger, he had been out of town during our whole visit. Surely he would want to have a voice in the selection of a colleague with whom he would have to work so closely and share so much. I never did meet him until after every detail had been settled. Over the years I must have given him many an occasion to wish he had at least been consulted before the die had been cast, but if he had any regrets, he never let me know.

Dr. Zollinger had a formidable reputation. Progressing through his surgical training program was a course in survival. The strong he alternately tolerated and supported, the weak he ground unmercifully into pulp. No one successfully challenged his authority. He was feared and respected by everyone, including all the professors in his department. His mastery of surgery was complete, and his standards so high that he was rarely satisfied. He placed a high premium on publication, believing that the number of scientific articles one had in print was an important index of one's worth. Every resident on his service was required to prepare at least one article for publication every year. Some had written many more. I had been in training for seven years and my second article, though accepted for publication, had yet to appear in print. Bill thought I might be able to overcome this handicap, but he wasn't at all sure.

Patty and I hoped to return to Columbus within a month to beard the lion in his den, and if successful, to begin to look for a house. From what she had seen during our busy first visit, she was as dubious about housing as I was about Dr. Zollinger. Before our projected return to Columbus the New England Surgical Society held its annual meeting in a hotel in Boston. Dr. Zollinger was invited to chair a panel discussion, and I crept into the back of the hall to catch a glimpse of the legendary ogre. The rumors had not been exaggerated. I watched in awe as he chewed up and devoured four of New England's leading surgeons. Secure in the anonymity of the darkened auditorium, the audience loved the effects of his acid tongue and rapier wit, but no one would willingly have traded places with a member of the panel.

When the carnage was over I spotted Dr. Zollinger huffing up the stairs from the men's room. Figuring that he probably felt as mellow at that moment as he ever would, I introduced myself and told him that I had been given an appointment to see him in Columbus in two weeks. He whipped out a little pocket calendar and said, "Good thing you mentioned it, because I won't be there."

"Well then," I replied, "I'd better talk to you now." It was going to be murder, but there was no use delaying it.

"I've heard of you," he said, "but I haven't heard much to impress me. Anyone can take care of patients. The question is, what else can you do? Can you teach, can you do research, how many papers have you written?" I could teach, I hadn't done any research, and I had written two papers.

"Christ!" he exploded, "only two papers, and you're thirty-four years old! Chances are you'll never amount to anything! I wouldn't walk across the street to encourage you to come to Columbus, but if you want to come, I won't stop you."

I beat a hasty retreat to the nearest phone booth to tell Patty before he changed his mind. Apparently Peter, aged three, overheard the conversation and understood the fact that we would soon have a new home in the Midwest. Patty overheard him telling the Hendren children next door that we were moving to "New-hio."

21

Last Days in Boston

When my residency ended Patty and I planned to pack up our belongings and send them ahead to a warehouse in Ohio while we spent our first real vacation with our children by the ocean. There were still a number of formalities to go through, such as obtaining a license to practice in Ohio. The trustees of the Children's Hospital would have to ratify Dr. Baxter's decision to appoint me to the hospital staff, and Bill would have to submit a letter on my behalf from Dr. Deterling to Dr. Zollinger, who in turn would need Dean Doan's approval to appoint me to the faculty of the medical school. There remained a slight chance that our plans to move to Columbus might fall through, but to all intents and purposes Dr. Zollinger's gruff acquiescence had settled the issue. No amount of additional training could have placed me in a better children's hospital. There weren't any. There I could develop a large practice, secure in the knowledge that whenever I was not available my patients would be cared for by interns and residents of the highest caliber, supervised by either Bill Clatworthy or Tom Boles who were both superb children's surgeons. The opportunities for teaching and research were essentially unlimited. I could not have been more fortunate.

Dr. Deterling was greatly pleased to have his first chief resident so splendidly situated. I happened to be in his office when Bill called him to ask for a letter of recommendation for me. Dr. Deterling had been my chief for only a few months and had had

far less contact with me than Dr. Child or Dr. Gross, but the letter had to come from him because he was my current chief.
Over the phone he was very complimentary about my ability to
care for patients, and he seemed to know more than I thought he
did about my performance as a teacher of medical students. The
conversation was going very well, from my point of view, until
Bill brought up the subject of my publications. I had failed to
call my two papers to Dr. Deterling's attention, but to my
surprise he told Bill that he was familiar with them, "and I
wouldn't be surprised if he were working on a third." My heart
sank. There was no way I could gather the statistics necessary
for a third paper before the end of my residency. Dr. Deterling
hung up the phone and dictated a fine letter of support, indicating that he would co-author my third paper and would do everything he could to get it accepted for publication. His secretary went off to type the letter, officially confiscating most of
my hard-earned vacation.

The Hendrens had been wonderful friends. Their four boys
were about the same ages as our children. "Bruddy" Hendren
and Jeff were particularly close, having done everything together since they were four years old. They were now almost
ten. Our Amy and Will Hendren had been less than two when
we moved to "Pill Hill" and couldn't remember having been
apart for more than a day or two in all of their young lives.
Hardy and I had worked together for only a few months before
he went to Massachusetts General and I to Boston City, and
though we both returned to Children's, our assignments there
had not overlapped. When we got together at home Patty and
Eleanor complained that all we talked about was surgery. We
did swap some pretty exciting stories; at least Hardy and I
thought they were exciting. Patty and Eleanor put up with our
tales of glory, ran our homes, raised our children without us,
and kept our spirits high. Eager as we were to get on with our
lives, losing the Hendrens as neighbors was going to be hard.

The same was true of King and Ann Browne, whose four children were part of the little gang. Dr. and Mrs. Hermann, who
lived between the Hendrens and the Brownes, were devoted sur-
rogate grandparents to them all. Our neighbors on "Pill Hill"
were destined to stay there for some time. Dr. and Mrs. Her-

mann talked occasionally about moving to an apartment when
they got older, but it was mostly talk. In their late seventies, they
were managing very well in the house that had been their home
for many years. King Browne was established in a law practice
in Boston and had no reason to move. Hardy, who had finished
his training a year before I did, was starting up the pediatric surgical service at Massachusetts General to which he would devote
his entire professional life. Massachusetts General was farther
from "Pill Hill" than Children's Hospital, but there wasn't much
traffic when Hardy drove to and from work, and the Hendrens
had decided to stay where they were, at least for a few years.
We wanted to sell our house to a family who would grow as
close to our friends as we had.

We had never sold a house before, and were blissfully unaware of how difficult it can be. Later we heard many horror
stories of having to support two mortgages for a year or more
while unfeeling real estate agents paraded hundreds of strangers
through an unsold house without producing so much as a nibble.
For us it was a cinch. George and Bunny Baker, who were
friends of all of us and especially close to the Hendrens, took
one look at our house and offered us a handsome price which we
didn't have to share with an agent. Everyone on "Pill Hill" was
delighted, and evidently the Bakers were well satisfied, for they
have lived in the house for more than twenty years.

The children watched as an army of movers packed their
books and toys into barrels along with our dishes and other
belongings. When they were done they had filled thirty-seven
barrels. We couldn't believe we had accumulated so many possessions. They started to load the barrels and furniture into a
cavernous moving van, but went home for the night with the
loading half done, leaving the van wedged in our tiny driveway.
Patty and I sat down amid the wreckage and poured champagne
into two borrowed jelly glasses to celebrate our twelfth wedding
anniversary. Behind us lay the last year of premedical school,
four years of medical school and seven years of postgraduate
training. How empty and how different these years would have
been without her, and how far short of the mark I would have
fallen had not this tender comrade been at my side.

The next day the van pulled away and I took a last walk

through the empty old house that had served us so well. The rooms seemed enormous without furniture in them. Even Peter's little room which I had paneled before he was born, the study in which I had never studied, seemed larger than I had remembered it now that Peter didn't live there anymore. I had expected this to be a nostalgic moment, but it wasn't.

We spent our vacation at a summer house on the shore about an hour and a half south of Boston. Patty and the children had a happy time on the beach while I commuted back and forth to the musty medical records library at Boston City Hospital to fulfill my obligation to grind out my third surgical article. Dr. Deterling was interested in jaundice, which has a number of causes in which surgery can be helpful. The research department of Johnson and Johnson, the baby powder people, gave me a grant of five hundred dollars which I used to pay an assistant librarian to help me, and together we pored over the medical records of seven hundred patients who had come to the hospital with jaundice. While she abstracted the data from the charts I read more than a hundred articles in the medical library and convinced myself that nearly every aspect of jaundice had been covered more than adequately. There was no use repeating a message that was already in print because no publisher would consider accepting it. There had to be a new wrinkle somewhere, but the more I searched the more elusive it seemed to become.

We completed our review late one afternoon and sat in our dusty cubicle surrounded by seven hundred data cards. We sorted them by sex. Nothing new there; jaundice affects men and women about equally. We sorted them by diagnosis; again no surprises. We sorted them by age and a curious fact emerged. A remarkably high percentage of the patients who came to the Boston City Hospital had not developed their jaundice until they were over seventy years old.

It was commonly supposed that cancer was the principal cause of jaundice in the elderly, and the articles I had read seemed to support this notion, most of them were written by people who worked in specialized institutions. I concluded that when a large group of totally unselected patients was considered, benign conditions such as hepatitis and gallstones outnumbered malignancy at every age. Even in our small group of people over ninety years old, cancer was not the leading cause. I felt the elderly deserved a more optimistic approach than they often received and that our data made a strong case for going all-out to help them. With the data to support the argument, I sketched out a plan for evaluating the elderly jaundiced patient, and Dr. Deterling joined me as co-author. It was not an earth-shaking paper, but he managed to get it accepted for publication, and in this unlikely fashion the last obstacle to my future as a pediatric surgeon was overcome.

Finding a new house in Columbus had been far more complicated than selling our old one. We had had very little time in which to look while I was still in training, and with the exception of Bill Clatworthy and Tom Boles we did not know a soul who could advise us. I knew that Jim Sayre, who had been a fellow resident at Boston Children's, came from Columbus, and at his wedding we had met his parents and his sister, Dixie Miller, who still lived there. They were more than willing to help us, and Dixie took on the project with a vengeance. She was convinced that we would want to live in Bexley, an "old" suburb to the east of the city. Having grown up in a New England house built in 1790, I was amused to find that an "old" house in Ohio was one built before the Depression of 1932. There were several of these to be bought, but they were all beyond our means. Despite Dixie's best efforts, and despite considerably more concern on the part of the leading Bexley real estate agent than we would have enjoyed without her influence, we were not able to find a house we could buy in Bexley.

Bill had a friend in the real estate business in Upper Arlington, where most of the people who worked at the university lived. He was sure that "Iccky" Wollam could solve our problem. "Iccky" knew of a house that would soon be on the market, and although it had not been listed for sale he persuaded the owners to sell it to us, provided they could continue to live in it until the new house they were building was completed. We loved the house, and bought it despite the fact that we could not find out when we would be able to move in. "Iccky" found us an interim house to rent. The builder had filed for bankruptcy, leaving it in the last stages of completion, but as temporary hous-

ing it would be perfect. Among the finishing touches he had
failed to provide were screens for the windows.

With our housing problem satisfactorily resolved and the
manuscript of my paper on its way to the publisher I settled
down to enjoy the remains of my vacation. The children were
completely at home in our house by the ocean and were brown
as berries from long hours at the beach. I didn't enjoy sitting on
the beach very much, but the swimming was good and the
fishing better, and we had great parties both on land and at sea
on Barbara and Larry Austin's boat. Labor Day was upon us before we knew it.

We spent the Labor Day weekend plowing toward Ohio, tow-
ing a U-Haul trailer behind us. Everything we owned that
wasn't in the warehouse in Columbus was in that trailer, and we
were so loaded down that the trip seemed endless. On the morning of our first day in our temporary quarters Belle Boles appeared on our doorstep to welcome us. She told us where the
schools and the market were and was the soul of hospitality and
helpfulness. After she had answered all the questions we could
think of she took a final look around the house and departed. In
a few minutes she was back with a present for us. Belle was as
observant as she was thoughtful. She had brought us a flyswatter.

Patty knew a lot more than I did about what the children
were going through. "When you move onto a new block," she
said, "your best pal is your bike." The children had been without
theirs all summer. The movers had given us a bunch of big red
tags labeled "KEEP FRONT" to tie onto objects we would want to
get out of storage as soon as we arrived in Columbus. The rest
would remain in the warehouse until we moved into our permanent home. As soon as Jeff and the girls returned from their first
day of school Patty loaded them into the station wagon and
drove to the warehouse to retrieve the bikes. When the doors
were opened there they were, three bicycles and one tricycle,
right at the very front. And way in the back, in who knew
which of the thirty-seven barrels, were the pedals.

22

Cynthia

President Eisenhower's second term in office was nearly over, and Harry Truman was chortling to himself because the Republicans had been responsible for the law that prevented Ike from serving a third term. Everyone in Massachusetts had been sure John Kennedy would defeat Richard Nixon, and what I had seen in Mayor Curley's hometown had done little to dim my respect for the power of the Democrats to elect whomever they chose. I drove up to the Children's Hospital and parked my car behind an abandoned old Cadillac. A great deal of rust showed through the faded pink paint. All four wheels had been removed. The first leaves of autumn were drifted against it, and on it someone had pasted a brand new bumper sticker reading, "Help Kennedy Stamp Out Free Enterprise!"

In addition to this refreshing political bias, the people of Columbus differed in other ways from those we had left behind. They were less reticent than New Englanders and far more gregarious. They were absolutely crazy about football. We had been accustomed to sitting in bleachers filled with students and their dates, with a few faculty members and loyal parents scattered among them. The people of Columbus flocked to the "Big Ten" games in such hoards that an Ohio State student was lucky to get a seat in a stadium that held eighty-six thousand people. Woody Hayes, who coached the Buckeyes, was perhaps the best known and most widely revered man in the whole state. As a topic of consuming interest, basketball was not far behind. No garage was complete without a basketball hoop. A Buckeye basketball game seemed to coincide with every social gathering, and when the starting whistle blew the television set took over the party.

New England was not exactly mountainous, but nowhere in New England did the fields stretch out in such endless flatness as they did around Columbus. Autumn in New England started on Labor Day, and the air was crisp and cool when the children went back to school. Summer seemed endless in Columbus, and when fall finally came, about the middle of October, the leaves did not turn scarlet and crimson. In winter it did not often snow very much, which was a mixed blessing. There were few snowplows and fewer people who knew what to do with them. Four inches of snow could paralyze travel in Ohio as effectively as two feet in the Northeast. The climate and geography combined to deprive the children of many outdoor pleasures to which they had been accustomed, such as skiing, skating, and hiking in the hills.

No one we met had apparently ever dreamed of going away to boarding school. There were none in Columbus, and only two private day schools in this city of more than a half million people. Children in these schools started in first grade and went through the twelfth in the same little group. Though they were supported by the same group of parents, who sent their daughters to one and their sons to the other, the two schools were as separate as separate could be. The trustees had discussed and flatly rejected any thoughts of coeducation or merger. Most of the men had gone straight from their local high schools to the vast Ohio State University, which offered them a broad range of educational opportunities without disturbing their constricted horizons. Many of the women, on the other hand, had been sent East to college, where they acquired husbands who followed them dutifully home to Bexley or Upper Arlington. The feeling that Columbus was the center of the best of all possible worlds was thick enough to cut with a knife.

In keeping with this concept, the people we met considered their Children's Hospital the best of all possible hospitals and gave it tremendous support. They were unanimously convinced that having been invited to come from Boston to join the staff I must be both brilliant and lucky. They were half right. I was very, very lucky.

Bill and Tom were waiting inside to show me around. After a quick tour of the wards we retreated to their offices, which were in a little blue house behind the hospital. A second desk had been moved into Tom's office for me. To Bill this had seemed the obvious thing to do, but had I been in Tom's shoes I would have resented the intrusion of a perfect stranger into my already cramped quarters. Tom gamely insisted that he didn't mind. In a few minutes they made me feel completely at home. Then they wished me good luck and announced that they were leaving for San Francisco. Should I have any questions, they assured me, they could be reached during the next ten days at the annual convention of the American College of Surgeons. I had been to one of these massive conventions and knew full well that the chances of reaching one of them in that milling throng of thirty thousand people were about equal to placing a phone call to a private on the parade ground at Parris Island. I had been at the Columbus Children's Hospital less than an hour, and I was on my own.

They could scarcely have made it to the airport before I had my first patient. He was a little baby, about five months old, whose pediatrician thought he had a tumor in his chest. He also had a temperature of one hundred and four. His chest x-ray was striking. His heart and left lung appeared normal, but the entire right side of his chest was densely opacified. If this were indeed a tumor, it would have been very bad news, but fortunately it was not. The dense shadow on the x-ray was caused by fluid surrounding the baby's lung and was simply drained away by inserting a large tube between the baby's ribs. Empyema, as the condition was called, was fairly common, especially in little babies. It resulted from pneumonia, usually caused by staphylococci. In the days before penicillin, empyema had been highly lethal. After penicillin was introduced the survival rate became much better for a while until large numbers of staphylococci developed resistance to the drug, whereupon the mortality went up again. As erythromycin and some of the newer antibacterial agents came into use, staphylococcal empyema again became manageable, though far from all the babies who contracted it survived. Perhaps it was beginner's luck, but this particular baby promptly recovered.

My next patient really did have a tumor. Her name was Cynthia, and she was a pathetically ill little girl just over five years old. When she arrived at the hospital she was pale, wasted, and feverish and had a persistent, hacking cough. Under her ribs on her left side I could feel a smooth hard mass midway in size between an orange and a grapefruit. Even when she took in as deep a breath as she could, the mass did not move at all. Her chest x-ray showed at least a dozen round, fluffy white shadows scattered through both lungs. These varied in size from somewhat smaller than a dime to about as large as a quarter. The lower borders of both lungs were obscured, indicating that they were surrounded by fluid which gravitated to the bottom of her chest when she sat up. When this fluid was drained away it was not the thick, malodorous creamy fluid found in empyema, but clear, straw-colored, and watery. When a small amount of it was spun in a centrifuge and the sediment examined under a microscope, it was found to be loaded with tumor cells.

The fact that the mass in Cynthia's abdomen did not move with respiration suggested that it was really not in her abdominal cavity but behind it. The peritoneum which lines the abdominal cavity is a shiny, slippery membrane that facilitates movement of the organs it contains. Inside the peritoneum high on the left side are the stomach and the spleen. Behind it is the left kidney with the adrenal gland sitting on its upper pole. Malignant tumors of the stomach are very rare in children, though unfortunately not at all uncommon in adults. Malignant tumors arise in the spleen far less frequently than they do in the kidney or the adrenal gland, especially in babies and small children.

X-rays of the abdomen usually show, as they did in Cynthia's case, that the left upper quadrant of the abdominal area is filled with a tumor which displaces the stomach and spleen to the right, but usually one cannot tell from looking at these initial x-rays which type of tumor the patient has. Often, by injecting a radiopaque substance into a vein one can get a pretty definite idea. The injected material, which contains iodine, is concentrated by the kidneys and is excreted in the urine. Before making its way down the ureters to the bladder this opacified urine fills the collecting spaces within the kidneys, and x-rays taken at this time indicate whether these spaces are distorted by a tumor arising within the kidney substance or merely displaced by a tumor which arises outside the kidney. Kidney tumors distort the collecting system; adrenal tumors displace it.

The series of x-rays using injected radiopaque material is known as an intravenous pyelogram, or IVP. Hundreds of these studies are made every year in all children's hospitals whenever a child is suspected of having a problem, benign or malignant, affecting the kidneys. In tumor cases an experienced pediatric radiologist can usually, though not always, distinguish between distortion and displacement. On Cynthia's x-rays distortion was obvious, indicating that the tumor almost certainly arose within the kidney. In her case the IVP showed another disturbing fact —the lower poles of her kidneys were joined together. The tumor did not cause this malformation, known as horseshoe kidney, but I felt it could make removing the tumor more difficult, as it might have allowed the tumor to spread directly to the other side. She could live a normal life with only one kidney, but she could not survive removal of both.

The common malignant kidney tumor of infants and children was described in 1899 by a Dr. Wilms. In 1960, when Cynthia's tumor was discovered, the survival rate was about 80 percent for babies under one year of age, but it was less than 50 percent for older children like Cynthia. No one knew for certain why this was so. Dr. Gross thought it might be because pediatricians examined babies more frequently than older children, or because mothers constantly handling and bathing their babies had a better chance to feel the tumor earlier, before it had spread. If it could be removed before spread occurred, cures were common. After spread occurred cures were very rare.

Spread of Wilms' tumors occurred in two ways. One was by rupture of the kidney capsule, allowing the tumor to extend beyond it. The other was by the process known as metastasis. Cells broke loose from the tumor, floated in the lymph channels toward the heart, and became trapped along the way in little nodules of tissue known as lymph nodes. If they broke loose in blood vessels, they floated directly to the heart and were pumped throughout the body. They might lodge anywhere, but they could only survive and multiply in locations where they found conditions suitable for growth. Different types of tumors had different preferences. Wilms' tumors found the lungs a particularly fertile area, whereas adrenal tumors preferred the bone marrow. Tracking down and identifying metastases is very important because if any of them are not subjected to effective treatment they will eventually kill the patient.

If the entire tumor can be removed before spread occurs, surgery alone can effect a cure. Had her tumor been discovered earlier, surgery might have been all Cynthia required. Now something else was desperately needed. Wilms' tumors were known to be somewhat more sensitive than normal tissue to the effects of x-rays. If sufficient x-ray energy was directed to the bed from which the tumor was removed a greater number of children survived than when this was not done. Occasionally metastases in the lungs could be eradicated by x-ray treatments, but not often. There was a limit to the amount of radiation the body could tolerate, and in general the wider the field of exposure the smaller the amount of radiation that could be used. Radiation of the whole body, which would ensure treating every single malignant cell, would be ideal if it were feasible, but invariably if enough radiation to kill tumor cells was applied to the whole body, it killed the child as well.

Dr. Farber had just published the first report indicating that chemotherapy could improve the survival of children with Wilms' tumors. The drug he used was very toxic. The dose was measured in micrograms, usually fifteen to twenty-five a day. There are thirty million micrograms in an ounce.

Despite the fact that metastases from Cynthia's tumor had spread far from their origin in the kidney, removal of the primary tumor was considered essential. The primary tumor was by far the biggest mass of malignant tissue in her body, and expecting irradiation and chemotherapy to eradicate it was asking too much. Surgery alone could not cure Cynthia. Surgery and x-ray therapy were very unlikely to do so, but perhaps with surgery, x-ray therapy, *and* chemotherapy she might have a chance.

Nearly all the factors known to diminish the chances for cure applied to Cynthia. She was five years old, four years older than the babies who had the most favorable outlook. Her lungs were filled with metastases which were almost invariably fatal, at least before the introduction of chemotherapy. She was wasted and anemic, and her temperature was nearly one hundred and four. I felt she should be given a few days of medical support before being operated upon. Certainly she would benefit from blood transfusions, and perhaps from antibiotics. It was not clear whether her fever was caused by the tumor, which was certainly possible, or by pneumonia. We never found out, because we gave her both chemotherapy directed against the tumor and antibiotics against the possible infection, but whatever the problem, she did improve.

After four days her temperature was almost normal, her hacking cough had subsided, and she obviously felt better. Coincident with the drop in fever and the blood transfusions her color had improved and her rapid, thready pulse had become slower, fuller, and stronger. Bill and Tom would still be away for almost a week, and much as I wished that one of them could be available to back me up, I did not feel I could justify delaying her operation until their return. I watched the anesthetist put her to sleep and embarked on a major operation I had seen but never done before.

It turned out to be much easier than I had anticipated. The lower poles of the two kidneys were not joined by the large bridge of kidney tissue I had expected, but by a broad flat band not much thicker than a leather belt. The right kidney appeared totally free of tumor, as did the connecting portion. The left kidney with its large, smooth mass came away easily, and when it was removed there did not appear to be any obvious tumor left in the gaping space behind the peritoneum. Inside the peritoneum all the organs appeared normal. With the tumor gone the abdominal muscles were lax and easy to close. For the first time I began to think Dr. Gross had been right. No amount of training could so thoroughly prepare me that I would never have to face the unknown in the operating room. Perhaps, as he had insisted, I had been a resident long enough. He had shown me how to remove a Wilms' tumor, and for that I was grateful to him, but I really felt that Dr. Child, with his passion for careful and thorough preparation of patients for surgery, had had more to do with the success of the first steps in Cynthia's recovery than anything Dr. Gross had taught me.

Cynthia brought me for the first time into contact with Bill Newton. Bill was many things to Columbus Children's Hospital, among them Pathologist-in-Chief, clinician, and hematologist. He was to become one of the best friends I ever had. As far as cancer was concerned, he filled in Columbus the role Dr. Farber filled in Boston. He supervised the use of the anticancer drugs. His plan for Cynthia, patterned after Dr. Farber's, called for five daily doses of the drug, actinomycin-D. She received the fourth dose on the day of her operation and the last the next day. Then we would wait, and if all went well, which we both felt would be highly unlikely, he would repeat the course of five daily injections in three months.

Having spent the last year of my training caring for adults, I had almost forgotten the marvelous power of recovery little children have. Cynthia was fully recovered from her operation in half the time I would have expected even a healthy young adult to require. We obtained a chest x-ray every other day, and Bill Newton and I watched the metastases in the lungs regress until in about three weeks all but two had disappeared. When these two small shadows stopped shrinking we sent her for daily radiation treatments. Instead of having to subject her entire chest to radiation the therapist could direct it through a "portal" only two inches square. Radiation, which when given alone had rarely cured a child with lung metastases, finished the job chemotherapy had so effectively begun.

Thirteen years later Bill Newton gave me one of my most cherished possessions, a large color photograph of a beautiful teenaged girl. It was taken the day before Cynthia graduated from high school.

23

A Benevolent Dictator

We had two offices. The one in the little blue house behind the hospital was used for all our work in administration, teaching, and research—activities that were to occupy a much greater share of my time and energy than I had anticipated. There were literally dozens of committees to direct various aspects of running the hospital. One investigated every infection to determine if the child could possibly have contracted it through some failure on the part of the hospital or some break in technique by a physician or nurse. There was a committee to run the operating room, another to run the laboratories. There was a committee to scrutinize the keeping of medical records. There was even a committee to advise the medical librarian on the purchase of medical books and journals. Some of these committees met for two or three hours every week. Medical students, interns, and residents passed in an endless stream through our teaching programs, and planning their conferences, teaching sessions, and ward rounds could easily have become a full-time job. Research projects began with preparing grant applications and proceeded through gathering and analyzing data to writing a final report suitable for publication or presentation at a national scientific meeting. It was not unusual for one of these reports to go through ten or twelve revisions before it was finally ready for release.

To help us with our paperwork, and to coordinate the scheduling of our many commitments we had a small secretarial staff headed by Delores Britt. I had had many telephone conversations with Dee before I left Boston, and instinctively knew I would like her. She proved even warmer and more helpful than I had hoped. Spread out on my desk the morning I arrived were all the official papers and application forms I would need, completely filled out, waiting for my signature. She had seen to the details of obtaining my license to practice in Ohio, a process that had taken almost three months even for someone who knew how to go about it. Dee was a godsend.

Because our contributions to administration, teaching, and research were important to the hospital we were provided office space and secretarial salaries for those purposes, but the hospital insisted that we maintain a separate office in which to see our patients. The office for patients was in a converted house on Bryden Road, a long walk but a short drive from the hospital. This little kingdom was Helen Crompton's world. So formidable was Helen's reputation as a tyrant that I approached her with some trepidation, but I soon found out that she had anticipated my arrival with equal anxiety, and we got off to a much happier start than either of us had expected.

Residency training provides no insight into how to conduct a practice. I knew absolutely nothing about the medical economic facts of life. I had never seen a medical insurance form. A young surgeon embarking on a private practice without an experienced medical secretary to help him must feel as hopelessly lost as a sailor at sea without a compass. Helen gave me to understand that I would have no problems at all, as long as I did things her way. Her way was usually a pretty good way, though not, as she invariably believed, the only way. She could be as stubborn as an ox.

She showed me the doctor's office. I expected to sit in this office with parents while I discussed their children's conditions and outlined my recommendations for treatment. This was not Helen's way. Parents were to be dealt with in the little examining rooms. Each of these had one chair for the mother to sit on, but none for me. Things would progress faster and more efficiently, she assured me, if I stayed on my feet and kept moving. Between each appointment I was to retreat to the office and dictate a short letter to the doctor who had sent me the patient while she explained to the parents when the operation would take place and what they should do in the meantime.

It was just as well, she remarked, that I knew nothing about insurance forms, because she handled all that sort of thing and I would never see one. I very rarely did. In order to fill out these complicated two-page forms all she needed from me were a diagnosis, the name of the proposed operation, and the surgical fee. I had no idea what to charge for an operation, but Helen had all the fees in her head. She insisted that I put them down in my own handwriting, not at all for her information but so that I would not cross her up by quoting a different figure to the parents.

For me to give a parent an appointment for an office visit was a cardinal sin. Helen made all the appointments. Parents could see me anytime they wanted, provided they wanted to come on a Wednesday afternoon. Otherwise, if they had not already selected a surgeon, they could see Tom on Monday afternoon or Bill on Friday afternoon. No surgeon was ever in the office at any other time. Once the parents had designated me as their surgeon they would see Bill or Tom only in an emergency. Bill had established this policy, but it was up to Helen to decide what constituted an emergency. There weren't many emergencies in her book. A few parents muttered that she bullied them unmercifully, but most seemed reassured by her self-confident and autocratic manner.

For the most part physicians referred children to the office without specifying which surgeon they wanted to operate on them. Helen was scrupulously fair in apportioning these patients among us, and this enabled my practice to grow much faster than it would have had I depended solely on word of my availability to spread gradually throughout the community. A few physicians had preferences among us, and Helen invariably bent over backward to respect them, but never once did she give me an opportunity to suspect her of playing favorites.

As my introductory visit came to an end Helen showed me the little waiting room. Children never come to a surgeon's office alone, as many adult patients do, but are always brought by at least one parent, often both. In addition, grandmothers seem to have a fascination for accompanying them, as do curious brothers and sisters. It doesn't take many patients to fill up a pediatric surgeon's waiting room. Helen informed me in no uncertain terms that she would appreciate my arriving promptly to start office hours on time. The idea of a waiting room crowded with patients waiting to see me was a new sensation, and Helen could see that I enjoyed the picture much more than she did. Because of my many commitments at the hospital I was often unavoidably late. Helen was always a pretty good sport about it, but she never allowed me to escape her pained and aggrieved look whenever it happened.

On the following Wednesday afternoon I returned to see my first patients in the office. The fact that Helen made the appointments worked to my disadvantage that day, and provided me a handicap I took two years to overcome. Two patients came to see me. Had Helen scheduled the second patient first, I would have been off and running, as he had an obvious hernia about which his pediatrician had thoroughly briefed the child's mother. The examination took less than two minutes, and the mother seemed to have no questions at all.

The first patient had constipation. It seems strange, perhaps, that a pediatric surgeon should concern himself with constipation, but scarcely a week went by without each of us seeing at least one constipated child. There is one cause of constipation in children that can only be cured by major surgery. This is known as Hirschsprung's disease, named for the Danish pediatrician who described it. The children with this disorder have an abnormal segment of colon and rectum which must be removed. It is necessary to be absolutely certain of the diagnosis before subjecting a child to surgery of this magnitude. Far more frequently the child is anatomically normal and can be managed by a simple regimen. The first step in differentiating these two groups of children is to take and evaluate a detailed history. By the time a pediatrician has despaired of solving the problem himself and has referred the child to a surgeon, the history has been complicated by a number of therapeutic attempts, some of which have appeared temporarily beneficial. It takes time to obtain and sort out all this information.

My first patient had acquired the habit of constipation after performing in a perfectly normal fashion for at least a year after birth. Thereafter constipation gradually came to dominate his life. The explanation was very simple. The colon is a long tube lined by a membrane whose major function is to reabsorb water. The intestinal content enters the colon in liquid form and is transformed into a solid stool as it passes from one end of the colon to the other. If the child repeatedly ignores the normal urge to defecate, as young children often do, the colon becomes gradually distended with retained fecal material and the muscle in its wall becomes stretched and loses its tone. A vicious cycle is set in motion. Distention leads to inability of the colon to empty itself, which in turn leads to further distention.

For a time laxatives appear to help, and for the occasional period of "irregularity," as the drug companies euphemistically call it, the use of a mild laxative may be appropriate. If used more than occasionally, laxatives soon become ineffective, producing crampy discomfort but not the desired result. Another product is tried, and then another, in a futile attempt to find one that works. Mothers become discouraged and frustrated and frequently resort to a self-defeating system of rewards and punishments. The child, who doesn't enjoy displeasing his mother, becomes equally frustrated and gradually becomes convinced that he is "no good."

The treatment of habit constipation is remarkably simple. The objective is to empty the colon of the bulky content it has gradually accumulated and allow it to shrink to its normal caliber. The muscle in its wall then regains its normal tone and becomes competent to handle the job it is supposed to do. The only satisfactory way to empty a chronically overloaded colon is with enemas. No medications or dietary measures can be expected to do the job. The fluid need not be irritating. Warm tap water with a little table salt added to it is very satisfactory. The appropriate ratio is one teaspoonful of salt to a quart of water. Enough of this warm salt water is used to promote evacuation without producing discomfort. It may take several days to empty the colon. There is no hurry. It took the child a long time to get into his difficulty, and he will not be cured overnight.

As soon as the colon is completely empty the child begins to feel better, and he and his mother may realize for the first time how much constipation had interfered with his sense of well-being. They both soon lose their initial distaste for the enema procedure and begin to cooperate in a spirit of confidence that at last they are on to a system that works.

The enemas are given only once a day, and always at the same time. It is helpful to give them immediately after a meal, as distention of the stomach with food triggers a natural reflex producing rhythmic contractions of the colon which give rise to the urge to defecate. The child has learned to ignore these contractions, but he can learn to take advantage of them. After the colon has been emptied the enemas are continued daily for at least two or three weeks regardless of whether or not spontaneous bowel movements occur. Then they are gradually withdrawn, skipping no more than one day at first. Once the child has been weaned from them they are used only when a reasonable effort has failed to produce a bowel movement.

It is essential to convince the parents of the harmful effects of rewards and punishments. Defecation is a natural process not to be compounded by attitudes of virtue or guilt. An adversary relationship between mother and child is neither necessary nor beneficial. The problem of constipation, like any other problem with which a child needs his mother's help, is best dealt with in a peaceful spirit of cooperation.

In about a half hour I had satisfied myself that the little boy in my examining room had habit constipation, and the mother had begun to believe that by following my advice she could succeed in relieving her son of this distressing and frustrating problem. Not a bad half hour's work I thought to myself. Helen thought otherwise. She concluded that I was terribly slow. The fact that I had spent less than five minutes with my second patient did nothing to dissuade her. For Bill and Tom she scheduled one patient every fifteen minutes. For me she insisted on allowing half an hour between appointments. It was two years before she relented.

24

Is This the Promised Land?

Before he left for San Francisco Bill had seen twin baby girls in the office with inguinal hernias. They were six weeks old, an age at which incarceration frequently occurs, and sure enough, before he returned one of the babies arrived in the emergency room with a loop of intestine trapped in her hernia sac. We gave her a little Seconal, and as soon as she had dropped off to sleep we wrapped her feet and ankles in soft sheet wadding and tied them to the bottom of her little crib. Then we elevated the foot of the crib on big wooden blocks so that she slept peacefully in a steep head-down position. Within an hour the trapped loop of intestine had slipped gently back into her abdomen. The emergency was over.

Helen had scheduled the twins' operations for the morning after Bill's return. Had this baby been my patient I would have advanced her operation to within forty-eight hours of her incarceration, knowing that once incarceration occurs it can happen soon again. But she wasn't my patient. The risk of waiting for Bill to return was not very great, but it was real, and I agonized over whether to take this small risk or to operate on another surgeon's patient. I knew full well the explosive fury I could expect should Bill not agree with my decision, but I concluded that whether he liked it or not, the right thing to do was to take her to the operating room. The anesthetists and the operating room nurses thoroughly understood my dilemma, but they kept their

opinions to themselves. The baby made a smooth recovery and
went home the next morning. Helen gave her mother an appointment to come to the office in two weeks. Helen didn't tell
me what she thought either. When Bill returned I told him with
great hesitation what I had done.

"Just right!" said Bill, to my great relief. "You're in charge of
our patients when we are away, and you have to do what you
think is right for them."

That is the way it always was. In Bill's and Tom's absence I
made many decisions, some much less clear than this one, about
what to do for their patients. When they returned they did not
always agree with what I had done, but they never second-
guessed me. They did the same for my patients when I was
away, and all of our patients benefited from this unwritten rule.

When the two weeks were up, the mother brought the baby
to the office, and of course she brought the other twin too. Tears
were streaming down her face as she carried them up the steps,
and both babies were screaming at the top of their lungs. I was
sure some dreadful disaster had befallen my operation and could
hardly wait for the mother to get the baby's diaper off. She was
so flustered she undressed the wrong twin. When my incisions
were finally unveiled they were two of the neatest, most cleanly
healed incisions anyone could ask to see. The tears, it turned out,
were caused by a cat which had crossed the road in front of the
mother's car. She had jammed on the brakes, sparing the cat but
catapulting both babies, each in her own little car seat, onto the
floor of the car. No harm had been done, and the three left the
office considerably happier than they had been on arrival. Helen
had been grave and sympathetic throughout the brief visit, but as
soon as they departed she burst out laughing. The ogre had a
sense of humor after all. Bill soon repaired the other twin's hernia, and Helen later reported to me that Bill's incisions didn't
look any neater than mine. I don't think she mentioned that observation to Bill.

I was surprised to find that I had an old friend among the pediatricians in Columbus. Will Fernald had been a fellow resident
during my first year at Boston Children's. If I had ever taken in
the fact that Will came from Columbus, it certainly had not
stuck in my mind. In those days I had never given any thought

to Columbus. I was amazed to hear his voice over the phone late one night.

"I understand you are covering for Bill Clatworthy," he said. "How would you like to operate on a baby with esophageal atresia?"

Every pediatric surgeon loves the challenge of esophageal atresia. Other surgeons never see it because it is rapidly fatal if not dealt with in the first few days of life. Atresia means complete obstruction of a hollow tube. In babies with esophageal atresia the esophagus is not only obstructed, but the two ends are usually not even connected to each other. The upper portion terminates blindly in a pouch located high up in the back of the chest. The lower segment, which is much narrower than the upper, turns forward and communicates with the lower end of the trachea, or windpipe. The communication is known as a tracheoesophageal fistula.

This abnormal arrangement poses several problems for the baby. He cannot swallow the mucous and saliva he produces, let alone breast milk or formula. Because the trachea is connected to the lower portion of the esophagus, air can be forced down into the stomach every time the baby cries. When he tries to relieve himself by burping, the air does not go up the full length of the esophagus to his mouth, but empties directly into the bottom of his windpipe. Often the regurgitated air is preceded by a jet of stomach juice which floods his lungs. Stomach juice is very corrosive and causes a chemical pneumonia, laying the groundwork for a serious pulmonary infection. Without prompt recognition and timely surgical intervention the baby cannot survive.

The conventional way to handle this lethal combination of malformations was to attack all of them at once by opening the chest, dividing the tracheoesophageal fistula and suturing the two ends of the esophagus together. This very major operation, which took from two to four hours, gave fairly satisfactory results provided the baby was not premature and had not been allowed to regurgitate stomach juice and develop pneumonia. If the diagnosis was delayed or the baby prematurely born, the operation was less likely to save his life.

Will had made the diagnosis early enough. The baby was only four hours old. His lungs were perfectly clear, but he weighed just under three pounds, less than half the weight of a full-term baby. The x-rays of his abdomen were somewhat peculiar in that there was the expected amount of air in the stomach and duodenum but none beyond. I thought this was unusual but attributed it to the fact that Will had made the diagnosis so soon after birth that the air had not had time to progress further. As we reviewed the x-rays together, neither of us recognized the true significance of what we saw.

Back in Boston Dr. Gross had always been at his very best when he operated on a tiny premature baby, but even his consummate skill and delicacy too often failed to bring babies like this one safely through so major an operation performed under emergency conditions. As he watched them succumb to an operation that was too long and too complex, Lester Martin had wondered if there might be a better way. As is often the case, the answer lay in analyzing the baby's problems separately, asking which of them truly represented emergencies and which did not. The baby's inability to swallow mucous and saliva did not constitute an emergency, as these secretions could be aspirated or wiped away by attentive nurses. With intravenous fluids the baby could survive for more than two weeks without being fed. Lester concluded that the emergency treatment should focus entirely on preventing air in the stomach from forcing stomach juice up the lower portion of the esophagus into the trachea. If this could be prevented immediately, the other problems could be dealt with one by one in a far less hurried manner.

Lester's plan called for the immediate insertion of a gastrostomy tube into the baby's stomach. This could be done in a few minutes through a small abdominal incision. With this tube in place air could leave the stomach at once, rather than remaining there until so much had accumulated that a burp was inevitable. Then in an orderly, unhurried manner the chest could be opened a day or two later with the sole objective of separating the lower portion of the esophagus from the trachea and closing its end. Now the gastrostomy tube could be used to feed the child, as milk could no longer reach the airway even if the child should try to burp or vomit.

The operation to close the tracheoesophageal fistula was far shorter and simpler than that required to join the two ends of the esophagus together. With regurgitation prevented, the baby could be allowed to grow almost indefinitely, until he was fat and healthy and able to withstand two or three hours of major surgery. Then the final objective could be achieved at little risk, and the gastrostomy tube subsequently removed.

Lester had convinced Dr. Gross of the logic of this multi-staged approach, and I had seen a few babies managed successfully in Boston in this way. As yet neither Lester nor Dr. Gross had published any reports about it, and babies in Columbus were still being managed in the more conventional way.

Hoping that I was not being viewed as a know-it-all, I announced that I proposed to put in a gastrostomy tube at once and leave all further surgery for later. The anesthetist was openly skeptical. Little did he know that I was just as sorry as he was that Bill Clatworthy was not there. It was well after midnight. With the baby lightly anesthetized I opened the abdomen. It was like arriving late at a wedding and finding that I had come to the wrong church. The abdomen was strangely empty. The stomach and duodenum were there, as were the liver and spleen, but beyond the end of the duodenum the entire intestine was missing. The baby had simply been born without it. No amount of chest surgery could equip him to survive without an intestinal tract. In fifteen minutes the brief operation was over. Had Will and I appreciated the significance of what we had seen on the x-rays, perhaps even this brief procedure might have been avoided, though it would have been hard to say for certain that the baby had no chance to live without opening the abdomen to make absolutely sure. Had I proceeded in the conventional manner, I would first have opened the chest and subjected the baby to a three-hour operation that had no chance of helping him. The skeptical anesthetist, who had been saved most of a night's sleep by my decision to do what Lester had taught me, became a convert, and by noon the next day word had spread throughout the hospital that the new young surgeon had remarkable judgment. Lester, who by that time was chief of his own service in Cincinnati, would have smiled had he known.

The next night Will called me again. "You won't believe it," he said, "but I have another newborn baby with esophageal atresia!" At Boston Children's we were used to seeing about twelve in a whole year. This must be the promised land, I thought to myself. Unfortunately, this baby also had an associated malformation which made his survival impossible. He was born with kidneys no bigger than the head of a kitchen match. I discovered this in the middle of the night when I opened his abdomen to put in a gastrostomy tube. Again a long, futile thoracic operation was avoided, but it was a tough way to earn Brownie points.

Will was very supportive in helping me talk with the young parents. The babies looked robust and healthy at first, sleeping peacefully in their little incubators with their gastrostomy tubes protruding from the little bandages on their abdomens. It was terribly hard to accept our statement that nothing could prevent them from withering away and dying. I have always been grateful, when tragedies like these occurred, if the family's own doctor could participate in these discussions. All too often the parents came from distant towns, and I and all of the other doctors who confronted them in their moments of anguish were total strangers to them.

25

Pyloric Stenosis

The clinical congress in San Francisco came to an end, Bill and Tom came home, and the flow of patients to my practice abruptly ceased. The pediatricians who had seemed so eager to avail themselves of my services reverted to their old habits and sent all their patients to the surgeons with whom they were familiar. I would gradually become busy enough, even when Bill and Tom were both on the scene, but for the moment I was mostly an observer. There was a lot to learn.

Bill and Tom took teaching very seriously and devoted much more time to it than Dr. Gross or even Dr. Child. My previous mentors, especially Dr. Gross, had relied heavily on the teaching efforts of their senior and chief residents, whereas Bill and Tom were more inclined to do it themselves. They were both excellent speakers, and their formal lectures to medical students and residents were models of clarity. The rapid turnover of students and junior residents made a great deal of repetition inevitable, but although they covered many of the basic subjects over and over, their presentations were always fresh and interesting, and I seldom came away from one of them without having learned something new.

The same was true of their daily ward rounds. Teaching was the sole objective of these rounds. Visits to parents and decisions concerning patient care were made at other times. Attendance by all students and residents was mandatory, and lateness was not tolerated. All patients were teaching patients; in this sense there were no "private" patients. Every mistake was criticized, no matter who made it. Some of the residents found Bill's constant stream of criticism hard to take. My position as a staff surgeon sheltered me somewhat from the direct fury of his blasts, but I smarted whenever he lashed out at a resident for a decision I had helped to make. A few of the residents seemed to thrive on his torrents of abuse. They knew instinctively that his only purpose was to achieve superb patient care and that because he was made the way he was, Bill simply did not know how to teach in any other way. He had a favorite saying to the effect that harbors are made safe for mariners not by recording prosperous voyages, but by charting the rocks and shoals that court disaster. Bill seldom had to call attention to the same rock twice, but he seemed to have a genius for uncovering new ones.

In the operating room neither Bill nor Tom had Dr. Gross' technical brilliance, but they were careful, gentle, and precise surgeons whose operations routinely yielded very good results. Some of their patients developed complications, as do some of every surgeon's patients, but very few of these complications could be attributed to errors in surgical technique. Like Dr. Child, they were both very finicky about little details of pre- and postoperative care that can often spell the difference between success and failure. The junior residents who came to the service from other hospitals were usually happy to go back when their tours were over, but later they almost always admitted that their pediatric surgical experiences had been among the highlights of their surgical training. The chief residents, who came with the objective of becoming pediatric surgical specialists, were as competent when they left as any who were trained in Boston.

Bill Bailey was chief resident when I arrived in Columbus. He called me one Sunday morning and with barely concealed surprise announced that there was a baby in the hospital whose parents had asked specifically for me. Until that moment every child I had cared for had come to me because neither Bill nor Tom was available. Today they were both in town. In fact, they were both actually in the hospital, but the parents wanted me. I tried to accept the call nonchalantly, but I don't think I fooled Bill Bailey. It was an exciting milestone.

Peter and Ellen had moved to Columbus at about the same time we had, and a friend had written me to ask that I help them find an obstetrician. I had met them at the motel where they were staying and given them a list of obstetricians. A month before this momentous Sunday morning Ellen had given birth to a robust baby boy.

He had appeared perfectly healthy and had gone home with his mother shortly after birth, eating normally and gaining about an ounce a day. After ten days he began to vomit, at first only occasionally, but soon after every feeding. The vomiting was alarming. It was not the normal gentle regurgitation of a little bit of formula that frequently accompanies a burp. The baby threw up most of every feeding with a projectile force that seemed to increase every time he vomited. What came up was the same white color as what had recently gone down, indicating that it did not contain bile. In his third week, during which he should have gained almost half a pound, he gained not a single ounce, and thereafter he actually lost weight because of the vomiting.

Vomiting seemed to be the baby's only problem. He did not appear to be in pain, and had no fever or other sign of illness. He was frantically hungry whenever a bottle was offered to him. He had good reason to be frantic, for he was starving to death. He had pyloric stenosis.

The pylorus is the gateway from the stomach to the duodenum. It regulates the rate at which the stomach empties, permitting a meal which has been consumed in a matter of minutes to enter the intestine gradually over one or more hours. Like the rest of the gastrointestinal tract, the pylorus is surrounded by muscle. Stenosis, or narrowing of the channel through the pylorus results from enlargement of the muscle fibers that encircle it. The process can be likened to the cooking of a doughnut. An uncooked doughnut is a slender circle of dough with a large hole in the center. As it cooks, the dough expands and the outer diameter of the doughnut enlarges while the hole in the center grows smaller. Five or six doughnuts laid one on top of another would resemble a pylorus, a cylinder with a canal in the center that grows progressively narrower as the surrounding wall thickens.

Why the muscle of the pylorus enlarges in this abnormal fashion is not known. The condition affects boys about four times as frequently as girls. It seems to affect first-born boys more frequently than their younger brothers, though it can affect several members of the same family. The incidence in babies is greater if one of the parents had pyloric stenosis in infancy, particularly if this parent is the baby's mother. It is more common in some parts of the world than in others, and considerably more common in caucasians than in blacks.

The condition is very seldom recognizable in the first week of life. Vomiting usually begins in the second, third, or fourth week after birth. Babies who do not begin to vomit until they are more than two months old practically never have pyloric stenosis. The baby's size at birth, which roughly parallels his gestational age, seems to have very little bearing on the age at which he begins to vomit. Babies who are born prematurely do not seem to develop the condition any later in post-natal life than full-term babies do.

These observations have given rise to all sorts of speculation as to the cause of pyloric stenosis. The fact that babies appear not to be born with it but develop it after birth suggests that if the cause were known the condition should be readily preventable. When all the speculation is boiled down, nobody knows the cause.

Fortunately, pyloric stenosis has become one of the easiest to cure of all the surgical conditions that affect babies. The mortality, which was about 50 percent at the time of World War One, has fallen to a fraction of 1 percent. The few deaths that still occur are usually not related to pyloric stenosis itself but to some other abnormality that happens to coexist with it.

The diagnosis may be difficult to make when the baby first starts to vomit, but it rapidly becomes easier as the days go by. Key features are the absence of vomiting in the first few days of life, the absence of fever or other sign of medical illness, the persistence of a voracious appetite, the absence of bile in the vomitus, and the fact that the vomiting is so severe that it causes the baby to stop gaining and ultimately to lose weight.

When the baby is completely undressed one can often see a slow rippling motion under the skin of his upper abdomen.

Large waves pass slowly from left to right as the baby's stomach contracts in an effort to move its contents through the narrow pyloric channel. The enlarged cylinder of muscle that surrounds the pylorus usually can be felt as a firm, movable mass resembling an olive within the upper abdomen. Nothing in the abdomen of a normal baby feels like it. With a characteristic story and a palpable pyloric mass the diagnosis is secure. Occasionally, x-ray studies are obtained after the baby has been fed a suspension of barium. The large slow gastric waves can be clearly seen on the fluoroscope, and with patience the radiologist can usually obtain a film at the moment a thin trickle of barium makes its way through the narrow pyloric channel. These x-ray findings are sometimes helpful, but pediatric surgeons find that as their experience in feeling the telltale mass increases their reliance on x-ray studies decreases.

For many years pyloric stenosis was treated without surgery, and a few authors reported considerable success with medical treatment. No one reported success rates as uniformly good as those obtained with surgery, and today it is recognized that it is far safer to operate on the babies than to hope that they will survive if treated medically. The superb results reported by the major pediatric surgical centers can be achieved only by carefully preparing the babies before taking them to the operating room. If the vomiting has gone on for many days, this preparation may take forty-eight hours or more. Even when the condition is recognized promptly there is no justification to rush the baby to surgery.

The repeated vomiting does more harm to the baby than simply to deprive him of the fluid and calories he would otherwise have absorbed from his feedings. Along with the ejected formula he loses large quantities of stomach juice which contains hydrochloric acid, sodium, and potassium. As these are lost from the stomach they are replaced from body stores, and as the vomiting continues these vital stores become progressively depleted. Before a baby can safely withstand anesthesia and a surgical operation a major share of these lost substances must be replaced, usually intravenously, at a rate at which he can safely assimilate them. Water and sodium can be replaced quite rapidly, but rapid administration of potassium is very dangerous, and overgenerous replacement can be as hazardous as failure to give enough.

The severity of each deficiency can be measured separately, but the over-all magnitude of the derangement can be appreciated by considering the baby's weight. Rapid gains or losses of weight are almost entirely due to gains or losses of water. Peter and Ellen's baby, who weighed about seven pounds at birth, should have weighed nine pounds at the end of his fourth week. Having stopped gaining and begun to lose because of the vomiting, he arrived at the hospital a full pound below his expected weight. His father, who weighed about 170 pounds, would have to lose twenty pounds in a single week to reach a similar state of dehydration.

The medical student who was assigned to the baby's case was thoroughly grounded in physiology and chemistry. He understood the metabolic problem and had plenty of time to follow and observe what we did to correct it. When the baby was finally brought to the operating room things began to happen so fast that he saw only about half the steps that were taken there to make the anesthetic and the operation safe.

He scarcely noticed that the operating room was almost too warm for comfort. It had been specially prewarmed. He did not see the rubber pad beneath the sheet on which the baby lay. The pad contained a series of channels through which warm fluid could be pumped during the operation to help keep the baby warm. He did notice that the anesthetist inserted into the baby's rectum a length of slender gray tubing leading to a large electronic dial. On the end of the tubing was a heat sensor so that the baby's temperature could be monitored continuously. Not only could a fall in temperature be detected at once, but the anesthetist could immediately turn on the thermal pad beneath the baby and raise his temperature again.

A tiny stethoscope was pasted carefully on the baby's chest over his heart. On his wrist, where the pulse is felt in adults, was a tiny electronic pulse sensor. The tubing through which the baby had received intravenous fluid during the previous twenty-four hours was still taped securely in place. Thus, the anesthetist was in a position to note any increase in pulse rate or fall in blood pressure that might suggest we had not given the baby enough fluid, and he was prepared to give more at any time.

The baby's skin was strangely dry and pink because he had been given atropine. Atropine dries the secretions in the respiratory passages. Without atropine the irritating effect of the anesthetic gases sometimes causes such an outpouring of these secretions that they interfere with the baby's breathing.

An even more important threat to a baby with pyloric stenosis is the possibility of accidentally drowning in fluid regurgitated from the stomach and aspirated into the lungs while he is under the anesthetic. Even though the baby had not been given anything by mouth for twenty-four hours he had continued to produce stomach juice, much of which had remained in his stomach because his pylorus was obstructed. A tube had been inserted into his stomach, but the tube necessarily was quite small, and it was dangerous to place too much reliance on the ability of this small tube to empty the stomach completely. Instead of putting the baby to sleep and then inserting a breathing tube in his windpipe, as is usually done in the absence of obstruction, the order of these steps was reversed. While the baby was still wide awake, with all his reflexes intact, the anesthetist put a laryngoscope into his mouth, visualized the vocal cords, and gently slipped the breathing tube between them. He quickly connected the tube to the anesthesia machine, turned on the anesthetic gas, and the baby was asleep in a few seconds. Inserting the tube while the baby was still awake seemed somewhat barbaric, but it protected him from aspirating any regurgitated stomach content into his lungs.

While all these preparations were going on Bill Bailey and I scrubbed our hands and arms for ten minutes and donned our gowns and gloves. As soon as the baby was asleep Bill painted his abdomen with iodine. We covered the baby with a plastic drape and made an incision about an inch and a quarter in length just to the right of his umbilicus. There was very little fat beneath the skin. The entire abdominal wall was only about a quarter of an inch thick. Beneath the three muscle layers, which we opened one by one, lay the thin gray peritoneum through which I could see the dark red liver moving up and down with every respiration. On opening the peritoneum and retracting the liver upward we saw our target, a firm gristly swelling at the terminal end of the stomach. By gently pulling on the stomach I could lift the swollen pylorus clear out of the abdomen. Blood vessels the size of pencil leads arose on its lower border and encircled it front and back, but they did not quite meet on the upper front surface. Here I could make an incision running the full length of the pylorus without cutting any of these blood vessels. The muscle felt more like cartilage than like normal muscle and split with an almost audible crack to expose a soft pliable pink layer beneath. This was the submucosa that, together with the mucosa inside it, lines the pyloric canal. We were careful not to perforate these layers but simply to allow them to pout out into the defect we had created in the encircling napkin-ring of gristly muscle. The obstruction was relieved. There was nothing more to do than close the incision in the abdominal wall. After all the preliminary preparations the operation itself seemed almost anticlimactic to the medical student. But not to me. It was the first operation I had ever done on a patient whose parents had chosen me to do it, and although I did it more than twenty years ago I remember it as clearly as if it had been yesterday.

The baby made a very smooth recovery, as almost all of them do, and within a week was starting to gain in a normal fashion. He soon made up for all his lost time and except for a barely perceptible scar on his abdomen appeared normal in every way. If a baby must have a life-threatening condition that requires surgery, pyloric stenosis is the one to pray for.

26

Surgical Teaching

When I started to work in Columbus fewer than two hundred surgeons in the United States were devoting themselves exclusively to pediatric surgery. As one of the acknowledged leaders of this little band, Bill Clatworthy received many invitations to speak at medical meetings. He considered this an important obligation and did his best to respond to as many requests as possible, but he could not handle all of them. Shortly after I arrived he had to decline an invitation from his good friend Dr. Tom Santulli to address the staff of the Columbia Presbyterian Medical Center in New York. Tom Boles couldn't go, and Dr. Santulli graciously accepted Bill's suggestion that he send me to represent him. The subject I was asked to discuss was congenital intestinal obstruction.

Congenital means present at birth. In most instances congenital obstruction is caused by a malformation, either an atresia, which is a complete block, or a stenosis, a narrowing so severe that practically nothing can pass through it. Occasionally, the intestine is not attached to the back wall of the abdomen in a normal fashion and is free to become twisted. In other instances, the bowel itself is normal but is filled with abnormal content that is so sticky and viscid that it cannot be expelled. In addition, there is a form of congenital obstruction in which the muscle fibers of the terminal end of the intestine do not contract and relax as they should because the nerve fibers that govern their action are not normally developed. Together the various forms of congenital intestinal obstruction occasion more than half of all major operations performed during the first week of life.

After working in Columbus for about six years Bill reviewed the records of all the obstructed newborns he had cared for. In keeping with his fascination for the rocks and shoals that court disaster, he concentrated his attention on the babies who had not survived. There were three main reasons why he had not been able to save them. These were prematurity, multiple malformations, and delay in diagnosis.

Babies who are born prematurely are not simply very small babies. They have many organs that are not sufficiently mature to deal effectively with the conditions they encounter outside the womb. This is particularly true of their underdeveloped lungs. Even in the absence of other problems, very early birth imposes a high mortality. If, in addition, a tiny baby requires a major operation before he can begin to eat, his chances for survival are severely limited. Little is known about preventing mothers from going into premature labor, and once it is underway there is no foolproof way to stop it without harming the baby.

Babies with malformations in their intestines sometimes have malformations in other organs as well. The intestinal problem may be amenable to surgical correction, but as in the case of my first two babies with esophageal atresia, the other malformations may not. Only a few measures were known to be effective in preventing malformations. Great care was taken to protect mothers from exposure to radiation early in pregnancy. The danger of contracting German measles in the first trimester of pregnancy was recognized, but there was no effective vaccine, and the only way a young woman could protect herself from this potential hazard was to expose herself deliberately before becoming pregnant to someone who had the disease. Genetic counseling could prevent some congenital abnormalities, but most forms of congenital intestinal obstruction are not genetically transmitted. All in all, preventing malformations was no easier than preventing prematurity.

A surprising 46 percent of the babies who died were not born prematurely and had no associated malformations. They simply were not recognized as being obstructed until it was too late to save them. Here was an opportunity to make real progress. The key was to alert all physicians caring for newborns—obstetricians, pediatricians, and family practitioners—to the early warning signs. These differ somewhat from the signs of obstruction in older babies, but once a physician appreciates their significance he has little difficulty in recognizing them.

The first is obvious before the baby is born. Sheltered in the womb, a baby is surrounded by a membrane known as the amnion which contains about three pints of fluid. The amount of this amniotic fluid is governed by the balance between the rate at which it is formed and the rate at which it is eliminated. If elimination is interfered with, the amount of amniotic fluid increases, producing a condition known as hydramnios which is easily recognized by the doctor who attends the delivery. One of the principal causes of hydramnios is inability of the baby to propel swallowed amniotic fluid through the upper portion of his intestine so that it can be absorbed. Only recently had it been appreciated that nearly half of the mothers with hydramnios deliver babies whose intestine is obstructed. When hydramnios is present appropriate steps to confirm the presence of obstruction can be taken within minutes after the baby is born.

The second sign is the presence of an excessive amount of fluid in the infant's stomach at birth. Virginia Apgar, a brilliant anesthesiologist at the Columbia Presbyterian Medical Center, documented this beyond question. She found that normal babies have less than half an ounce of fluid in their stomachs when measured before they are first given anything to drink. The finding of more than an ounce or an ounce and a half in the stomach at this time almost invariably signifies intestinal obstruction. The fluid is in the stomach because it cannot be pushed farther down the intestinal tract. The finding can only be made by passing a small tube into the baby's stomach immediately after birth, a maneuver which many obstetricians and pediatricians had not been accustomed to perform.

The third sign is vomiting. Vomiting is common when tense and apprehensive mothers begin to feed their new babies, but it is distinctly unusual in nurseries when newborn babies are fed by relaxed and experienced nurses. Since most of the malformations causing obstruction are located beyond the point in the duodenum at which bile enters the intestine, the vomitus of obstructed babies usually contains bile which gives it a green color similar to that of a pool table cover.

The fourth sign is abdominal distention. A few babies with abnormal bowel content are actually distended at the moment they are born, but in the majority the telltale sign of abdominal distention cannot be recognized until the baby is several hours old. The abdomen becomes distended because the baby swallows air that he cannot pass. The degree of distention depends on the location of the obstructing abnormality and the rapidity with which air is swallowed. If the malformation is toward the upper end of the bowel the resulting distention will be minimal, since air can only enter the part of the bowel that lies above it. If the obstruction is near the rectum, massive distention of the abdomen will eventually occur if not prevented. Many newborn babies are wide awake and alert in the hours immediately after birth and tend to swallow air rapidly. Sometimes medications given to ease the mother's discomfort during the last stages of labor pass across the placenta and narcotize the infant so that he sleeps for several hours and swallows air much more slowly.

Virginia Apgar is also credited with pointing out the fifth sign. She carefully documented the time at which hundreds of babies passed their first bowel movements and found that this almost always occurred before they were twenty-four hours old. The content of the colon at birth is called meconium. The ancient Greeks noted that babies seemed to become more active after they expelled this substance which they erroneously believed kept them sleepy in the womb. They knew the soporific effect of the poppy plant, from which they derived the name. Normal meconium is greenish black because of the presence of altered bile pigments. The colon of a full-term baby contains about six ounces of this dark material. Failure to pass any of it within twenty-four hours of birth, or passage of a scanty amount of material which does not contain bile, is distinctly abnormal and warrants investigation even in the absence of any other sign of trouble.

It is important to recognize that no baby can be expected to manifest all of these danger signals. Only obstructing abnormalities located near the upper end of the bowel give rise to accumulation of excessive amniotic fluid, while only those near the terminal end can cause great abdominal distention. Diagnostic steps must be taken promptly when the first sign is recognized, regardless of which of the five it may be. Feedings are withheld and the baby protected from vomiting and aspirating fluid into his lungs. X-ray studies are obtained on an emergency basis.

The swallowed air contrasts sharply with fluid within the bowel and with the bones and soft tissues of the baby. Since x-rays are negatives, air appears black while more dense substances appear gray or white. Only one bubble of air within the abdomen, the one in the stomach, is normally wider than an adult's thumb. Any other large air bubbles are contained in portions of intestine which have become dilated before the baby was born by futile attempts to force fluid past a long-standing obstruction. If only a few large bubbles are present the obstructing abnormality is located in the upper portion of the bowel. If the x-ray shows many distended loops of bowel the obstruction is near its terminal end.

Careful introduction of a suspension of barium into the baby's rectum can be very helpful in sorting out the various causes of obstruction and may indicate the urgency with which operation is required. If the barium enema shows that part of the colon is misplaced within the abdomen, the baby must be operated upon at once, even in the middle of the night, because the intestine is twisted and death will ensue if it is not untwisted promptly. If the entire colon is in its normal position but very tiny in caliber, the obstruction is in the small bowel above it. Sometimes the barium enema looks entirely normal but x-rays taken several hours later show that the baby has retained most of the barium instead of expelling it as other obstructed babies do. This usually means that the nerve fibers in the terminal portion of the colon have not developed normally. These babies have Hirschsprung's disease and require a colostomy so that the abnormal portion of the bowel can be bypassed. They will require a major operation, such as the one developed by Dr. Swensen, when they are several months old. In other babies an obstructing plug of meconium can be washed out of the colon by an experienced pediatric radiologist. To operate on a baby who can be cured by this simple procedure would be a tragic and entirely preventable blunder.

X-ray examination of obstructed babies is not very time-consuming. It is seldom necessary to spend more than an hour in the X-ray Department, but the importance of obtaining an accurate diagnosis before operating on a baby cannot be overstressed. A surgeon without a target cannot expect uniformly good results. Bill must have said that a thousand times on his ward rounds.

The operations needed to relieve the various forms of congenital intestinal obstruction have become standardized and are not very complex, though they require utmost delicacy in their performance. In the absence of very premature birth or lethal associated malformations, the great majority of obstructed babies can be rescued from certain death and go on to lead perfectly normal lives—if they are recognized in time.

That was the essence of the talk I gave in Bill's stead at the Columbia Presbyterian Medical Center in the fall of 1960. Bill worked tirelessly to help me prepare it, raising in advance every question he could anticipate my being asked and making sure I knew the answers. The talk was well received in New York. More important, the exercise of preparing it served as an introduction to my role as a surgical teacher in Columbus. Over the years I have given hundreds of talks like this one to interns, residents, medical students, and groups of physicians.

Because of the extensive teaching efforts of many pediatric surgeons an early diagnosis of congenital intestinal obstruction is rarely missed today, and very few babies are deprived of a fighting chance to get well. Usually that is all they need. One of the greatest rewards of surgical teaching is watching a resident surgeon sort out the possible causes of obstruction and perform the appropriate life-saving operation on a baby only a few hours old. It was always a thrill to do it myself, but it became an even greater thrill to watch a younger surgeon do it and know that I had taught him.

27

Roses and Visitors

We had been waiting for a call from Mr. Edwards. Before we moved to Columbus we had bought his house on condition that he and Mrs. Edwards could continue to live in it until their new home was built. One evening Mr. Edwards called to say that they were moving soon and that if we would come over he would like to show us around. I envisioned a tour of the furnace and fuse boxes, but that was not what Mr. Edwards had in mind. He wanted to introduce us to our new roses.

There were 174 of them, nearly all different. There was the large, pure white Peace variety with a fully open rose measuring four inches across. There was a small bush with almost coal-black blossoms. No one, Mr. Edwards remarked wistfully, had been able to raise a pure black rose. I wasn't sure why anyone would want to, but obviously he did, and he had come very close. There were roses of every shade of red, pink, orange, yellow, and lavender. He called each of them by name, recalling the difficulties he had had with this one and the contest he had won with that. Realizing that I could not possibly remember all of them, he had drawn a plan of the eight beds and carefully written down the name of every bush.

I began this tour as a dubious observer, but before it was over I had become a convert. He had opened my eyes to a whole new world of infinite variety and incredible beauty. I did my best to follow his instructions and spent many pleasant hours spraying and adding just the right amount of fertilizer. We had glorious roses, but they never looked quite as lush and healthy as they had under Mr. Edwards' tender care.

A day or two after we moved in we received an invitation to membership in the American Rose Society from the president, who turned out to be none other than Dr. Zollinger. Dr. Zollinger was Mr. Edwards' most competent and fiercest competitor. It was rumored that he had bested Mr. Edwards in a recent contest by feeding his roses out-dated blood from the University Hospital blood bank, but I never was able to confirm the story.

In our new home at last, we settled the furniture we had stored in the warehouse and set about unpacking the thirty-seven barrels. In the next to last of them we found the long-lost pedals. As I bolted them in place on the children's bicycles I felt for the first time a feeling of permanence in Ohio. We were barely settled when our first overseas visitors arrived.

The idea that children can be cared for best in hospitals designed and organized to meet their special needs became prevalent in the United Kingdom earlier than in the United States. The same was true of the notion that surgeons might obtain better results by devoting themselves exclusively to children than by dividing their attention between children and adults. The two concepts go together, it being easiest for surgeons to concentrate on pediatric surgery when they work in large children's hospitals. London, Liverpool, Edinburgh, Montreal, Toronto, Melbourne, Sidney, Brisbane, and Perth all have major children's hospitals, most of them older and much larger than ours. Working in them are pediatric surgeons with enormous experience from whom we in America have much to learn. The long distances that separate these children's hospitals give the surgeons a feeling of isolation that they try to overcome by infrequent but extensive travel. Bill availed himself of every opportunity to invite them to visit Columbus.

The "mother" hospital for many of our British, Canadian, and Australian colleagues is The Hospital for Sick Children on London's Great Ormond Street. It has a long tradition of excellence in child care and many loyal supporters, both lay and professional. Charles Dickens made fund-raising speeches for this venerable institution, and James Barrie assigned to it the royalties from *Peter Pan*. Graduates of its surgical training programs can be found in every corner of the empire, from where many loyal alumni make the long pilgrimage to London every four or five years. Having satisfied their yearning to return to their Alma Mater, a number of them set forth for America, bringing with them the latest ideas from Great Ormond Street and a wealth of information from their own surgical centers. We looked forward to their visits, for they were delightful guests. Having come a great distance, they usually stayed longer than American visitors, giving us a better chance to get to know them.

First to arrive was James Mason-Brown, Surgeon-in-Chief of the Children's Hospital in Edinburgh. He was so modest and self-effacing that it was difficult to appreciate the prominence to which he had risen. He failed to mention it, but Bill had learned that he had recently been elected president of BAPS, the British Association of Pediatric Surgeons. He gave us several lectures and participated with us in a number of operations. His comments revealed him to be a careful, thoughtful surgeon who had followed his patients meticulously and knew in great detail the results of the many operations he had performed. He was aware of new ways to attack old problems, but he reminded me of Dr. Chamberlain in his caution against discarding sound methods in favor of promising new ones that were not yet thoroughly tested. His outstanding attribute was common sense, and few men were more richly endowed with this precious commodity than Jimmie Mason-Brown.

His wife, Louie, came with him. She was an enthusiastic traveler who found much to delight her in what we considered a rather mundane Midwestern city. Patty had the brilliant idea of inviting Tony and Dixie Miller to dinner with the Mason-Browns, and they became fast friends. Tony owned a unique piece of property way to the north of Edinburgh. It was situated next to a castle belonging to Britain's queen mother, and Tony had bought it for a price that would stir the envy of the most scottish Scot. On Tony's land were the remains of a very ancient castle and a more "modern" one in which one could live quite comfortably in summer time. Louie and Dixie had many good

times together at the castle and in Edinburgh, and still corre-
spond more than twenty years after first meeting in our home.

Next to come were Mr. and Mrs. Russell Howard. (Surgeons
are called "Mr." in the British Commonwealth.) Mr. Howard
was Surgeon-in-Chief of the Royal Children's Hospital in Melbourne, an institution nearly three times as large as any children's
hospital in America. He was especially interested in thoracic
problems and had a huge experience in esophageal atresia and
pectus excavatum, or funnel chest. The largest published series
of children with funnel chest in this country numbered about a
hundred. Mr. Howard reviewed for us his personal experience
with more than nine hundred cases. He cautioned us against the
temptation to operate on children until they were at least five
years old, as he had had fewer recurrences in children over this
age. He emphasized the benefits of physical therapy, showing
with many excellent photographs the improved results he obtained when the children were taught breathing exercises before
being operated upon and were carefully supervised for a number
of months afterward.

He had been troubled, as we had also, by a few children with
esophageal atresia in whom there was so long a gap between the
upper and lower segments that the two ends of the esophagus
could not be sewn together. He had very convincing x-rays
showing that he had been able to lengthen the upper segment by
gentle stretching done repeatedly for many days before the operation was performed. Apparently he had been lucky in the selection of the first babies for this procedure. We were seldom
able to duplicate his results, and some years later he wrote to say
that he had become discouraged by the few instances in which
his technique seemed to work in Melbourne.

Mr. Howard was a collector of fine silver, which he said was
very scarce in Australia. He showed us a magnificent sterling
teapot that he had acquired on his trip, and it took only one look
to assure us that his expertise extended beyond surgical matters.

The Australians had been leaders in reducing the death rate
from a rather common problem of early childhood. While Mr.
Howard was with us a child with typical symptoms was admitted to my care. He was a beautiful, healthy seven-month-old
baby who had never been sick for a day in his young life. A few

hours before he came to the hospital his mother noticed that he seemed momentarily to be in great pain. He suddenly stopped playing, turned pale, drew up his legs, and screamed. She was about to call her pediatrician when he abruptly returned to his former self, playing happily with his toes as if nothing had happened. There seemed to be absolutely nothing wrong with him. An hour later it happened again. His eyes took on a glassy stare, he lost interest in his surroundings, drew up his knees, and screamed. His mother ran to him and picked him up but could not comfort him. It was as if he were surrounded by an invisible shield that she could not penetrate. He was entirely preoccupied by whatever was hurting him. Again she reached for the telephone only to see him relax and quickly return to his former happy self. This time she did call the pediatrician who recognized over the phone that the baby had an intussusception.

Intussusception is a telescoping of the intestine. Typically, a portion of the ileum, the part of the intestine nearest the colon, slips inside the part of the bowel beyond it. The enveloping segment contracts, producing a spasm of pain lasting from a few seconds to a minute or more. Then the bowel relaxes and the pain goes away. The trapped intestine does not slip back again but gradually progresses until two to four inches or more are surrounded. Brief, intense episodes of pain recur with gradually shortening intervals, reminiscent of labor pains. Many, but not all of the babies vomit.

The blood vessels supplying the trapped intestine become engorged, causing that portion of the bowel to swell. When the baby relaxes between attacks of pain gentle palpation in the upper abdomen reveals a smooth cylindrical mass that is said to feel like a sausage—the big German kind. Being more familiar with bananas than German sausages, I have always felt the mass to resemble the middle third of a banana from which the third on each end has been discarded. The mass usually is not tender to touch. It is firm but not hard, and is somewhat movable within the abdomen.

Examination of the rectum is not remarkable shortly after the onset of the pains, but after a few hours this maneuver produces bloody mucous when the examining finger is withdrawn. Sometimes a "currant jelly" stool is passed spontaneously, but more often the rectum must be examined to find it.

Once established, intussusception is almost always an irreversible process that ends in death if not recognized and treated. The Australian surgeons had few secrets as far as treatment was concerned. The reason for their superior results was that they had systematically educated all the physicians in Australia to recognize the condition early and refer the children immediately for surgical treatment. We in America were beginning to do the same for infants with congenital intestinal obstruction.

Surgery gave excellent results when intussusception was recognized early and the babies carefully and vigorously prepared for their operations. The telescoped intestine cannot be pulled back into the normal position, for pulling merely makes the surrounding bowel hug it tighter. By slow and gentle compression the trapped intestine can usually be pushed back the way it came. Occasionally it will not budge and must be removed along with the bowel that holds it. The baby can spare the involved segment of intestine and grows normally without it, but complications are fewer if resection is not necessary.

When the diagnosis is in doubt a barium enema usually gives conclusive evidence. The radiologist and surgeon watch on the fluoroscope as the barium suspension travels retrograde up the colon until it meets the intussusception. Here it abruptly stops with the end of the column of barium indented by the tip of the intussuscepting mass. Every pediatric radiologist has had the exciting experience of seeing the mass move slowly backward under the pressure of the barium suspension, even to the point of complete reduction of the intussusception. There were a few reports in the medical literature of cures using plain enemas, but these were doubly dangerous. Without the fluoroscope and the barium the doctor could not see when he had effected a complete reduction and thus did not know when to stop. In addition, if he exerted too much pressure and perforated the bowel, he had no way of recognizing what he had done in time to save the child from death from overwhelming peritonitis.

Dr. Mark Ravitch, working at the Baltimore City Hospital, did an exhaustive study of intussusception which he reported in a classic monograph. He studied the amount of pressure normal intestine can withstand, as well as the amount of pressure required to reduce most intussusceptions. Largely as the result of his work, the use of carefully controlled barium enemas replaced operation as the initial step in treating children with intussusception.

The pressure exerted by the enema fluid is controlled by the height of the fluid's container above the patient. The higher the container, the greater the pressure, since the fluid flows in by gravity. Dr. Ravitch established the safe height to be no more than 36–42 inches above the x-ray table on which the baby lies. This relatively low pressure is sufficient to reduce between 70 and 80 percent of the intussusceptions commonly encountered. As long as this pressure is not exceeded, the danger of perforating the intestine is essentially nil. Perhaps higher pressures would reduce a few more and spare a few babies an operation, but the risk of perforation is too great.

After carefully preparing the baby for the operation he would need if reduction by barium enema were not successful, Mr. Howard and I took my little patient to the X-ray Department. Under the fluoroscope we watched the column of barium suspension make its way up the descending portion of the colon on the baby's left side. Behind the stomach it turned and proceeded from left to right until it stopped midway across the transverse part of the colon where the leading end of an intussusception is usually met. The baby had been sedated with morphine and slept throughout most of the procedure. Nothing happened for a minute or two, as more barium suspension flowed in behind the obstructing mass. Then it began to move, very slowly at first, and then rapidly down to the cecum in the right lower quadrant of the abdomen. The cecum is the part of the colon to which the small intestine attaches. Here the barium column hesitated for a moment, and then there was a sudden rush of barium into the terminal part of the small intestine. The intussusception almost certainly had been completely reduced, but just to be sure we kept the baby in the hospital for about twenty-four hours. He had no more pain and next morning was ravenously hungry. He went home at noon and I never saw him again.

The ease with which a barium enema can reduce an intussusception correlates roughly with the duration of symptoms, but there are many exceptions. Some children whose diagnosis has been unrecognized for as long as several days can still be relieved by the method while others cannot, even if the duration of their symptoms is less than six or eight hours. Nevertheless, on the average the sooner barium enema reduction is attempted the more likely it is to succeed.

Because children who are not relieved by barium enema must be operated upon at once, it was our practice to prepare every one of them ahead of time for the operation we hoped they would not need. This entailed cross-matching blood in the blood bank, giving intravenous fluid, and placing a tube in the stomach to empty it. Intussusception is, after all, a form of intestinal obstruction. Some surgeons routinely give antibiotics to all children with intussusception, others only if operation is needed. This careful preparation may prove excessive in some cases, but the unpredictability of success in the X-ray Department has validated repeatedly the wisdom of taking the trouble to do it every time.

The small group of children who do have to be operated upon are handled in one of two ways. In about two thirds, the intussusception can be reduced manually by gently squeezing the bowel back to its normal position. In about a third the trapped intestine is so tightly held that it cannot be reduced safely and the involved segment must be removed.

Occasionally an anatomic abnormality, such as a polyp in the intestine, may serve as a leader, dragging the intestine in after it. These are rare. In fully 95 percent of children with intussusception no anatomic abnormality can be found to explain its occurrence. Experience has shown that barium enema reduction practically never succeeds when one of these anatomic abnormalities is present, so that all children who have them are highly likely to be operated upon. The fear expressed by Dr. Gross in his book that many of these abnormalities might be overlooked unless all children with intussusception were operated upon has been shown to be unfounded.

Regardless of the method used to reduce the initial intussusception, a few children experience recurrences. For a time it was predicted that recurrences would be seen more frequently in children who were not operated upon for the first episode, but they are not. Either way, about 97 percent of children are relieved of a single intussusception and never have another. An occasional child experiences multiple attacks that can only be stopped by removing a small portion of intestine. In twenty years I never saw one, though I heard of one or two.

Except in the case of the very few children with anatomic abnormalities, the cause of intussusception is unknown. For some obscure reason it is more common in boys than in girls. One study in England seemed to show that a virus might be involved, but other studies failed to confirm this. The incidence varies widely from one part of the world to another, suggesting that diet or cultural factors may play a part. In Columbus we saw, year after year, about one child with intussusception for every five or six with appendicitis. The condition has been seen as early as the day of birth, and a few instances are noted in every decade of life, but the vast majority of patients are children between the ages of three months and two years. Finding ways to prevent it must await indentification of its cause. Speculation abounds, but so far the cause of intussusception has eluded everyone.

28

Appendicitis

Although our patients ranged in age from a few minutes to twenty-one years, they were not evenly distributed over this span. Half of them were less than two years old. The youngest were infants with congenital malformations who came to us directly from the delivery room in which they were born. There were many older babies with hernias, pyloric stenosis, intussusception, and malignant tumors. There were also a number with burns and other injuries, some of which resulted from parental abuse or neglect. In addition, there were always a few with relatively uncommon conditions, including some very young children with appendicitis.

In the children over two years old we saw injuries, including many burns, appendicitis, malignancies, and a number of congenital malformations, including hernias, which had not been recognized or required treatment earlier in life.

Our patients were divided by age into two groups or "services" called "under two" and "over two." This allowed the interns and residents to form two teams, each responsible for a limited and clearly defined group of patients. It also made it easier for the staff to supervise them and to assume responsibility for the relatively large number of children whose parents either had no preference or did not know how to select a surgeon. Teaching and supervision of patient care were assigned on a rotating basis in which Bill shared equally with Tom and me and with two general surgeons who devoted a limited amount of their time to pediatric surgery.

One of these general surgeons was Dr. Warren Harding, a distant relative of the former President. For my first tour "on service" Bill teamed me up with Dr. Harding, giving us responsibility for the children over two years old. We were a happy combination. Dr. Harding was looking forward to retirement; I was just beginning. I had had more formal training in pediatric surgery than he, but he had the practical experience I lacked and was a wise and conscientious teacher. We liked each other and worked very harmoniously together.

Being assigned to the over-two service did not preclude my caring for infants who were referred to me, and one night I operated on a newborn baby with congenital intestinal obstruction. The baby recuperated nicely but was not ready to go home when his mother was released from her maternity hospital. She visited him frequently in his little crib and spent many hours in the hospital every day. One afternoon she treated me to a great surprise.

Dr. Harding and I had just finished our rounds and stood talking together when she chanced to pass us in the hallway. I thought she gave Dr. Harding a quizzical look as she walked by, but his back was turned and he did not notice her. After he left she approached me and asked, "Wasn't that Dr. Harding I saw you with just now?" I replied that it was and she went on, "We think he is the most marvelous man. He looked after our older child here in the hospital for nearly a year when she was burned. How he got her through I'll never know, but he saved her life. You ought to see her now, so healthy and happy! Dr. Harding is just wonderful."

Perhaps I should have nodded in silent agreement and let it pass, but the temptation was too great. "Well," I said, "why didn't you ask Dr. Harding to look after your new baby?"

"Oh," she said, "we just take who they give us." Had her first encounter with Dr. Harding ended in tragedy, I could have sympathized with a wish to deal with a different surgeon, but in the circumstance she described I found her reply utterly incomprehensible. I have thought about this strange response many times over the years, but I have never understood or ceased to wonder about it.

In children over two years old appendicitis is the most common condition requiring abdominal surgery. We looked after about a hundred and fifty children with appendicitis every year. Like intussusception, appendicitis begins with pain, but in nearly all other respects the two entities are a study in contrasts.

The ages of children with the two conditions overlap, but children with intussusception tend to be much younger. Mothers of children with intussusception can pinpoint almost to the second the time when the pain begins, whereas the onset of pain in appendicitis is more insidious. At first the pain of appendicitis is vague and poorly localized. When children are asked where they first appreciated pain they do not point to a spot with one finger, but tend to rub the whole center of the abdomen. In contrast to the strikingly intermittent pain of intussusception, that of appendicitis tends to be constant.

Most children vomit, as do most with intussusception, though it is my impression that vomiting usually is more prominent in appendicitis. Virtually all lose their appetite, and some who do not vomit indicate that they think they would feel better if they could. It is distinctly unusual for hunger to persist very long after the onset of appendicitis.

In the early stage fever is absent or the temperature elevated only a degree or two. Children whose temperature reaches 103 or 104 degrees very soon after the onset of pain usually have something other than appendicitis. The white blood cell count rises moderately, with a preponderance of young cells, suggesting that the body is mobilizing its defenses against a bacterial infection. Very low white blood cell counts are unusual and suggest that a virus, rather than appendicitis is the cause of the problem. A few children with appendicitis have essentially normal white blood cell counts.

If they are examined very early, there may be little to suggest appendicitis, and every experienced pediatrician has sometimes missed the diagnosis in this early stage. Gradually the vague, diffuse discomfort becomes more intense and shifts from the center of the abdomen to a point below and to the right of the umbilicus. When the abdomen is now examined a discretely localized area of tenderness is found at this point.

Loss of appetite, nausea, vomiting, and pain are seen in a great number of children, most of whom do not have appendicitis. The order in which these symptoms appear is very important. If pain occurs late, after the other signs of intestinal upset are well established, the appendix is usually normal. Abdominal pain as the *first* symptom is appendicitis until proven otherwise. Often the only safe way to be sure is to hospitalize the child for a brief period of observation. Most children and parents accept this advice, fully understanding that the trouble may subside without need for an operation.

In order to allay apprehension and facilitate evaluation of the abdomen, sedation with a medication such as Seconal is often useful. Sedatives like Seconal do not diminish organic pain or mask tenderness as do opiates like morphine or Demerol. Morphine is a wonderful drug, but it cannot be used to facilitate the evaluation of abdominal pain. Sedation is generally not advisable at home but should be carried out in a hospital under the supervision of the surgeon who will remove the appendix if that becomes necessary.

With appropriate sedation and frequent examination appendicitis soon becomes clearly recognizable. The pain does not subside, and tenderness in a localized area in the right lower part of the abdomen persists and becomes more prominent. When it is established that the child has persistent localized tenderness, the appendix should be removed without further delay. There is a chance that a normal appendix will be removed, but the risk to the child is far less than the danger of procrastination.

I have performed hundreds of appendectomies and doubtless forgotten many of my patients with appendicitis, but one I remember very well. Perhaps it was because she was another surgeon's daughter. Shirley was a pretty blue-eyed blonde with a touch of red in her hair who came home from school with a stomachache and did not want her supper. At first I could not be sure whether her abdomen was truly tender or whether she was merely apprehensive at being examined by a stranger. When her father palpated her abdomen with the gentleness only a father can muster I became convinced. She winced whenever he touched a spot below and to the right of her navel. She knew she faced an operation if she betrayed the fact that it hurt, but she could not help herself. I knew well enough the importance of listening to mothers. This time I'm glad I paid attention to a father.

She needed little preparation for the simple operation she was about to undergo. Now that the decision to operate had been made, we gave her an appropriate dose of morphine which made her feel much better. We started an intravenous infusion and placed a plastic tube through her nose into her stomach. Vomiting and aspiration of stomach contents into her lungs was a complication to be avoided at all cost. With these simple steps accomplished we took her to the operating room less than an hour after she had walked, slightly bent over, into the hospital.

The anesthetist put her to sleep by injecting sodium pentothal into the intravenous tubing. Pentothal by itself is not a satisfactory anesthetic when the abdomen must be entered because in safe doses it has little muscle-relaxing effect. As soon as she was unconscious a mask was placed over her face and the pentothal supplemented by a mixture of oxygen and halothane. Halothane is an almost ideal anesthetic. Its action is very rapid, and it is quickly eliminated when no longer needed. It does not smell awful and is not explosive. It produces good relaxation of the abdominal muscles which makes the surgeon's job much easier than when they are tense and rigid.

The appendix in young children tends to lie higher in the abdomen than in adults. An incision placed low enough to be covered later by a bikini would be cosmetically ideal, but a higher one is usually safer. As long as the incision runs in the direction of the natural skin folds the resulting scar will be minimal. Vertical or slanted incisions that cross these natural skin lines result in much more prominent scars. The incision I made in Shirley's abdomen began about half an inch below and two inches to the right of her umbilicus and extended laterally from that point for about three inches. Beneath the fat lay the outer muscle layer of the abdominal wall.

The fibers of this outer layer run downward and medially, paralleling the prominent skin crease that separates the abdomen from the leg. Opened in this direction the muscle retains its greatest strength. The middle muscle layer is much thicker and has fibers that run at right angles to those of the outer layer. The fibers of the inner layer run transversely. Opening each layer in the line of its fibers produces a short "gridiron" incision which is very strong when healing. This incision gives limited access to the abdomen, and much longer ones must be made for many operations, but for appendectomy a small "gridiron" incision, if placed high enough, is ideal.

When the three muscle layers were opened and their edges separated with retractors the peritoneum lining the abdominal cavity came into view. Beneath it lay the cecum, the first part of the colon. The cecum resembles a mitten lying in the right lower quadrant of the abdomen with the fingers pointing down and the thumb pointing centrally. The thumb represents the terminal end of the small intestine, and from the cuff of the mitten the colon ascends on the right side of the abdomen toward the liver. There it turns and crosses from right to left toward the spleen where it turns again behind the stomach and descends along the left side to terminate in the rectum. The appendix arises at the point on the mitten within which the tip of the index finger would lie. When healthy it is somewhat more slender than a finger and varies from one to four or five inches in length. The location of its base is constant, but the tip can point in any direction, as can the hand of a clock. On cross section it resembles the rest of the intestine, having a shiny outer membrane beneath which are two muscle coats and the submucosa and mucosa, or lining layer. The narrow channel within the appendix comes to a blind end at the tip, so that any material that gets into the appendix can only leave by returning to the cecum from which it came. As long as this material is liquid or soft no harm is done, but a mass of firm fecal material may become stuck in such a way that the muscular wall of the appendix cannot extrude it. The first pain of appendicitis is believed to result from vigorous muscle contraction as the appendix attempts to empty itself. Many children who have appendicitis report that they have briefly experienced this type of pain before, suggesting that on prior occasions the appendix has successfully relieved itself of similar obstructions. The obstruction may be facilitated by kinking of the appendix or by narrowing of a part of the channel, but why some people develop appendicitis while most do not is largely a matter of conjecture.

If obstruction persists, inflammation accompanied by infection follows, beginning in the lining layers and extending to the outer surface. At this time the pain shifts from the middle of the abdomen to the right lower quadrant, localized tenderness becomes prominent, and the diagnosis of appendicitis can be made.

We grasped the cecum and drew it gently out of the abdomen, followed by a short length of small intestine and the base of the appendix. This part of the appendix was normal in caliber and a healthy pale pink, but about an inch from the base it abruptly widened and from there to the tip, a distance of about two inches, it was engorged and fiery red. We divided the blood vessels of the appendix, crushed its base with a clamp and tied it securely. The appendix was amputated and the short stump covered over by folding it into the wall of the cecum and securing it with sutures. The cecum was returned to the abdomen and the incision closed layer by layer. That was all there was to it. After the operation was over we opened the appendix and found the central canal obstructed by a fecalith, an almost stony hard ball of fecal matter.

Usually children with this simple form of appendicitis are in the hospital three or four days, but since Shirley's father was a doctor and her mother a nurse, I let her go home the morning after her operation, and except for a single postoperative visit I never saw her again.

Children try very hard to please their doctor, and sometimes he has to take what they say with a grain of salt, but I have heard so many children insist that they felt better immediately on awakening from an appendectomy than they did before being put to sleep that I have come to believe them. Apparently, if made carefully and handled gently, the incision in their abdominal wall doesn't hurt very much when they wake up. I gave them morphine before their operations, for which they always seemed grateful, but very few of them wanted morphine afterward.

29

Rupture of the Appendix

Recognized early and treated by prompt appendectomy, appendicitis is among the simplest of surgical diseases to manage successfully. The cure rate is 100 percent, and since children have only one appendix, recurrences after appendectomy do not occur. Complications are rare and deaths almost unheard of. But appendicitis is relentlessly progressive, and if the diseased appendix is not removed within a few hours, the surgeon is faced with a very sick child who now has a number of complex problems. Recovery from operation is slow and stormy, serious complications frequently occur, and a few children still die from advanced appendicitis.

Shirley had hardly danced out the front door of the hospital when Sandra arrived in the emergency room. She was about two and a half years old and obviously gravely ill. Her story was as follows. Four nights earlier she had become whiny and fussy and picked uninterestedly at her supper. Perhaps because she was so young her mother did not appreciate that pain was a prominent part of her illness. She later admitted that she thought appendicitis only affected older children. At any rate, she was not alarmed and put Sandra to bed where she spent a restless night. She vomited two or three times before morning and would not touch her breakfast. Her pediatrician was called. He advised keeping her in bed and giving her liquids to drink. He would see her later if she did not improve.

He did see her about four that afternoon. She lay quietly on his examining table, curled up in a ball, and was irritable and miserable whenever she was disturbed. Her abdomen appeared somewhat tender all over without a specific point of maximum tenderness. As her mother described it, vomiting seemed to be the most prominent feature of her illness. During the day her temperature had risen to 103 degrees. She was a fat little girl in whom it would be difficult to recognize the onset of abdominal distention. There was a "virus" going around, and Sandy looked very much like a number of children her doctor had seen with a self-limited form of gastroenteritis which lasted two or three days. He advised continuing bed rest and encouraged her mother to continue offering fluids whenever Sandy would accept them.

Reassured that her doctor was not worried, and that Sandy was not expected to make a rapid recovery, her mother took her home, canceled her bridge game, and settled down to make her as comfortable as possible while the intestinal upset ran its predicted course. The next day Sandy seemed no better but did not appear appreciably worse. Her mother did think her abdomen was perhaps a little larger than usual, but she was not sure of this. Sandy was not able to keep down the liquids that were offered to her and gradually lost interest in trying to swallow them.

On the fourth day, when she was worse rather than better, her doctor sent her to the hospital. She resisted all attempts to examine her and cried whenever any part of her body was touched. I gave her a dose of Seconal, and in about twenty minutes she dropped off to sleep. Now she did not move when I touched her arms, legs, or chest, but whenever I touched any part of her abdomen she opened her eyes, cried out, and pushed my hand away. When I listened to her distended abdomen with my stethoscope I heard none of the gurgling noises the intestine usually makes. Except for the transmitted sounds of her breathing her abdomen was completely silent. She had peritonitis.

In the early hours of her illness her appendix had become obstructed and subsequently inflamed. The inflammation had spread to involve all layers of her appendix, proceeding more rapidly than it would have in an older child, perhaps because its wall was so thin. A portion of the wall had given way, allowing millions of bacteria to pour out into the abdominal cavity where normally not a single bacterium can be found. Like older children, Sandy had an omentum, a filmy apron of fat that hangs down from the stomach and transverse part of the colon. The omentum of adults and older children has a marvelous tendency to adhere to an inflamed appendix and help to confine the spread of infection. But in babies and small children the omentum simply is not long enough to reach the appendix and thus she was denied this valuable protection. Unencumbered by the omentum, the bacteria were free to spread to all parts of her abdominal cavity producing an infection which before the advent of antibiotics was nearly always fatal in young children.

Despite the most effective antibiotics known, peritonitis still kills children, and is especially likely to do so if the source of the bacteria is not eliminated. In Sandra's case the source was the hole in the wall of her appendix. Removing the appendix was essential, but the real emergency was not to operate upon her at once but to prepare her so that the operation would not kill her.

She had several major problems. Despite the fact that she had not communicated it very well she had been in severe pain for four days. Now that we had made a diagnosis we gave her a generous dose of morphine.

She had a serious infection so widespread that it could not be cured by operation, though the source of continuing contamination could be removed. The peritonitis that results from rupture of the appendix is usually caused by more than one species of bacteria, as many types normally inhabit the cecum and appendix. Most of them are sensitive to the combination of streptomycin and penicillin. We gave Sandra these two drugs before, during, and after her operation.

Because she had vomited repeatedly and taken in very little fluid over the past four days she was severely dehydrated. The abdominal infection had caused an outpouring of fluid into her peritoneal cavity, making the dehydration even worse. We gave her liberal amounts of intravenous fluid and plasma.

Her abdomen was greatly distended. The intestine had responded to the inflammation and infection by losing its propulsive force. For this reason the air which she continued to swallow was unable to make its way through the intestine but remained trapped within it. As she swallowed more air the distention became progressively worse. There was little that could be done to remove the air already trapped in her intestine, but at least we could prevent more from accumulating. We placed a tube through her nose into her stomach and attached it to a little mechnical pump so that swallowed air would be sucked up out of her stomach before it had a chance to go through the pylorus into the intestine.

A final problem, resulting both from infection and from dehydration, was fever. The margin of safety is very small when little children with high temperatures are subjected to anesthesia. Rather than risk catastrophe it is safer to delay operation a few hours until intravenous rehydration, aspirin, and external cooling with sponge baths bring the temperature down. As the fever drops and fluid depletion is partially restored the pulse begins to slow. On admission Sandy had a temperature of 104 degrees and a pulse rate of 156. Three hours later these were 101 and 124. She looked and felt much better. It was tempting to delay the operation even longer in hopes of further improvement, but experience has shown that little is gained by further procrastination and that often if the operation is delayed, the child's improved condition deteriorates again.

The interior of Sandy's abdomen could only be described as a malodorous mess. After aspirating away large amounts of foul smelling purulent fluid I located the appendix, nearly divided in two by a huge hole in its wall. Fortunately, the fecalith that had initiated the miserable train of events was still in the appendix. Otherwise we would have had to make a careful and possibly extensive search for it among the inflamed and distended loops of intestine. If left behind it would serve as a nidus of continuing infection. After removing the appendix we placed a "cigarette" drain into the depths of her pelvis, leaving the upper end protruding from her incision. Cigarette drains resemble cigars, being as big around as an adult's finger. They are tubes of very soft thin rubber stuffed with gauze. Their use reduces but does not completely prevent the formation of abscesses within the abdomen and pelvis as the child recovers.

Sandy was in the hospital for almost a month. Her convalescence was marked by several days of high fever and very slow return of bowel function, requiring the suction tube to remain in her stomach for about ten days. During all this time she could take nothing by mouth and required a constant intravenous infusion. She required regular doses of morphine for several days. Nevertheless, she was spared a number of the postoperative complications we sometimes saw in children with ruptured appendices. She did not require a second operation to drain an abscess. She did not return a few months later, as several less fortunate children did, with intestinal obstruction due to adhesions which may form as the inflammation subsides. The one complication we still cannot be sure she will not have is sterility. A number of girls who have had peritonitis in their early years develop such severe scarring of their fallopian tubes that an egg cannot make its way toward the uterus to be fertilized.

With unruptured appendicitis so simple a disease and ruptured appendicitis so formidable, one would think that parents and physicians would rarely fail to recognize the disease in its early and easily treatable form. The fact is that very little improvement has been recorded since before the Second World War. In general, the younger the child, the more rapidly the disease progresses. In children less than two years old the appendix has almost always ruptured before a doctor ever sees them. To remove an inflamed but still unruptured appendix from a three- or four-year-old is the exception rather than the rule. Thereafter it becomes more common, perhaps because the disease runs a slower course, perhaps because older children more effectively alert their parents to their early symptoms.

Long after Sandy's stormy battle with appendicitis Bill Clatworthy made a study of children whose appendices had ruptured. Half of them might have gotten to a surgeon before rupture occurred had the first physician to see them recognized that they had appendicitis. The other half were not seen by any doctor until after their appendices had ruptured. Thus the blame for missing the diagnosis appears to be shared about equally by parents and physicians. It is easy to point fingers but not easy to suggest ways to improve this record. Appendicitis continues to baffle parents and frustrate the physicians and surgeons who care for their children.

30

JP

Until Bill Clatworthy came in 1950 neither Columbus nor any other city in Ohio had ever had a pediatric surgeon. Today there are six in Columbus and at least fifteen in the state. The population has increased, but not faster than that of the nation as a whole, and while the number of families is greater, the number of children per family is smaller. There really are not many more children in Ohio today than there were thirty years ago.

There is a lot more that can be done now to help children who need surgery. In part this is due to earlier diagnosis and advances in surgical technique, but in large part it is due to other factors. These include a host of new antibiotics that help to control infection, greatly improved anesthesia, and better understanding of intravenous fluid therapy, blood transfusion, and nutrition. Pediatricians specializing in the care of newborns and premature babies have been enormously helpful. Among their important contributions has been the skillful use of respirators that can support children for long periods of time, respirators without which many fragile little babies would tire and die because they could not sustain the work of breathing after major operations.

Most newborns are operated upon by surgeons who specialize in child care. The same is by no means true of older children, nor is every newborn operated upon by a pediatric surgeon. Pediatric surgeons are the general surgeons of childhood. General surgeons have been defined as those who do what is left after the specialists have done their work. Prominent among the surgical specialists of childhood are neurosurgeons like Drs. Matson and Ingraham, orthopedists, plastic surgeons, heart surgeons, ear, nose, and throat specialists, and urologists. The tendency for a few members of these surgical specialties to concentrate exclusively on children developed later than it did in general surgery, but now there are many pediatric neurosurgeons, pediatric orthopedists, and so on. Children have benefited greatly from this willingness to concentrate on their special needs.

Pediatric surgeons interact with all of these specialists, and sometimes the boundaries are rather fuzzy, particularly in dealing with injuries. Neurosurgeons naturally care for children with severe brain injuries, and neurosurgeons are skilled at repairing injured nerves in the arms and legs as well. But most nerve injuries are accompanied by injuries to skin, muscles, tendons, blood vessels, and often bones or joints. Therefore, plastic surgeons, orthopedists, and pediatric surgeons all have experience in repairing nerves, and probably fewer than one injured nerve in ten is repaired by a neurosurgeon. Urologists are specialists in operating on kidneys, but many children with kidney injuries also have injuries to other organs. Clearly, surgeons in many disciplines must work together harmoniously if shattered children are to be given the best opportunity to survive. Jurisdictional guidelines are helpful, but ultimately it comes down to mutual respect and unselfish cooperation.

It was this spirit that pervaded the Columbus Children's Hospital and made it a happy place in which to work. Among the many specialists with whom I shared responsibility, two stand out as best exemplifying this cooperative spirit. Martin Peter Sayers was an exuberant and enthusiastic extrovert, a national leader in the generation of pediatric neurosurgeons who followed Drs. Matson and Ingraham. His capacity for work far exceeded mine. In fact, perhaps his greatest fault was reluctance to admit that he couldn't continue forever to handle all by himself the growing flood of children with neurosurgical problems who came to Children's Hospital. The pediatric urologist was a quieter, more introspective man named John P. Smith. "JP" and

I cooperated in a number of adventures and in the process became the best of friends.

One night while JP was out of town I operated on a little boy who had been hit by a car. Jimmy arrived in the emergency room only a few minutes after the accident, but already he was pale and thirsty with a rapid pulse and a falling blood pressure. His abdomen and left flank were very tender. It seemed clear that he was losing blood, probably from a ruptured spleen. The spleen lies in the left upper part of the abdomen just in front of the left kidney. When the spleen is injured by a blow or a fall the left kidney is often injured as well.

We gave Jimmy intravenous fluid and blood which slowed his pulse and raised his blood pressure. We knew he would need an operation to prevent further bleeding, but we had at least a few minutes in which to study him for evidence of other injuries. He soon produced a urine sample for us, and it was red with blood. I performed an intravenous pyelogram, a series of x-rays exposed after injecting Hypaque into a vein in his arm. Hypaque contains iodine and when concentrated and excreted in the urine casts a dense shadow on the x-ray film outlining the spaces within the kidneys that contain urine.

The shape of the shadow on the left side of Jimmy's x-rays did not seem just right to me, but his left kidney contained so little Hypaque that I really could not be sure whether it was normal or not. We took him to the operating room, opened his abdomen, and found the expected ruptured spleen which we removed without difficulty. There were no other injuries within the abdomen, but the left kidney, which lay behind the lining of the abdominal cavity, was surrounded by a large blood clot. Instinct told me not to disturb this clot, and therefore I did not get a good look at the injured kidney. I closed the abdomen and took Jimmy to the recovery room, hoping that I had done the right thing. He had an uneventful convalescence, for which I was grateful, but I was plagued by a lingering feeling that rather than knowing how to deal with his injured kidney I had just been lucky.

JP and I studied the x-rays the next day with the help of Tom Frye, one of our senior radiologists. We all agreed that the intravenous pyelogram was not of sufficiently good quality to give an accurate assessment of the injury to the kidney. I reviewed the steps I had taken in obtaining the films. It was a conventional study done in the conventional way. We repeated the intravenous pyelogram using the same technique and the result, if anything, was less revealing than my original. There had to be a way to get better kidney x-rays.

In addition to Children's, Tom worked in another hospital in which the patients were adults. He told us that in studying adults he was beginning to use a new technique known as infusion pyelography which seemed to yield much better pictures than conventional intravenous pyelograms. He showed us an article from the *Journal of Radiology* in which the authors described their technique very clearly but did not mention using it for children. We were sure that the amount of Hypaque they recommended for adults was far too much for little children. JP and I decided that we should attempt to modify the technique of infusion pyelography so that it could be used safely in children of all ages. Our chief resident, Marc Rowe, now Chief of Surgery at the Children's Hospital of Pittsburgh, became an enthusiastic collaborator.

Conventional intravenous pyelograms are sometimes inadequate because during the time the x-ray films are being exposed the kidneys are excreting urine too slowly. As urine containing Hypaque enters the collecting spaces within the kidneys it is carried away to the bladder before enough has accumulated to fill them. In infusion pyelography the rate of urine flow is increased by giving a rapid injection of fluid. When this is done the spaces in the collecting system of the kidney fill completely, but it is necessary to give several times the usually recommended dose of Hypaque in order to produce a dense shadow. For adults the authors recommended five ounces of Hypaque, about seven times the standard dose. Convulsions and permanent brain damage can result if safe limits are exceeded. Neither Marc, Tom, JP, nor I knew the safe maximum for children.

Don Hosier, our pediatric cardiologist, injected large quantities of iodine-containing materials to obtain x-rays that outline the cavities within the heart. He gave us a schedule of what he considered the maximum safe doses for children of different ages and said he had never had toxic effects when he stayed within these limits. With these figures to guide us, we worked out the technique of infusion pyelography in infants and children. We induced a rapid urine flow by adding to a large amount of Hypaque an equal amount of sterile saline solution and injecting the diluted mixture over the course of a minute or two. This was a sizable amount, comparable to injecting more than half a pint of fluid rapidly into the vein of an adult.

Using this new method we studied children with all sorts of kidney problems. As soon as we had performed infusion pyelograms in enough children to be confident that our technique was safe and effective we published our results. This simple exercise, for which Marc Rowe and Tom Frye deserve much credit, resulted in an improved method of studying kidney problems in children which is now used throughout the world.

Use of infusion pyelography was the first step in trying to improve our treatment of children with kidney injuries. We now knew how to obtain much better x-rays, but we still were not always sure what to do with the information they provided. JP and I reviewed the records of seventy-eight children treated for kidney injuries during the preceding few years. Many of them had done well, but we identified a number who had obtained less than optimal results. We looked for the rocks and shoals that had courted disaster.

A few children appeared in retrospect to have been operated upon too soon after injury. Kidneys that we thought might have been saved appeared to have been removed because the surgeon had great difficulty in controlling bleeding from hundreds of tiny blood vessels in the freshly broken kidney tissue. On more than one occasion the surgeon had decided that quickly removing the kidney was less risky than unduly prolonging the operation in order to bring the vexing bleeding under control. The children who had been operated on one or two days after the accident seemed to have fared better, presumably because at that time bleeding was easier to control.

On the other hand there were a few children in whom the need for operation had not been recognized for a week or more. Sometimes the surgeon had appeared unsure of what constituted a need for operation. Sometimes the conventional intravenous pyelograms were of such poor quality that we could not recognize the need for operation even in retrospect. These children did not do well, for by the time they finally got to the operating room a virulent infection had set in, surrounding the injured kidney with a pool of pus in which it could not heal. All of these kidneys, which we felt might have healed if given a better chance, had been removed.

Many adults live in good health for years after removal of one of their kidneys, but if we could save all or a major part of a child's kidney we felt we should try to do it. After all, a healthy ten-year-old can be expected to live more than sixty additional years. Our review suggested that about four of every five children with kidney injuries do not need surgery, but that one of the five will benefit from a well-timed operation aimed at conserving as much kidney tissue as possible. In addition to describing how to obtain better kidney x-rays, JP and I set out to define as clearly as possible how to recognize the one child in five who should be operated upon.

The kidney has four basic parts. These are the kidney tissue, the capsule that surrounds it, the urine-collecting system in the center, and the main blood vessels that nourish it and bring waste products to it. If only the kidney tissue and the capsule are injured, operation is almost never needed, but if the collecting system or the blood vessels are disrupted, surgery is usually required. The infusion pyelogram can give important information about the status of each of these components.

The most frequent injuries are contusions, or bruises, of the kidney tissue. They usually result from falls, athletic injuries, or automobile accidents. The child has pain and tenderness in the upper abdomen and flank and a variable amount of blood in the urine. Sometimes the urine is dark red; sometimes the presence of blood is only detected by chemical tests or by seeing a few red blood cells under a microscope. If the child is unconscious as a result of the accident, the presence of blood cells in the urine may be the only clue that one of his kidneys has been injured, since unconscious children cannot give evidence of pain.

The infusion pyelogram shows that the collecting system, the series of urine-containing spaces in the center of the kidney, is compressed. Kidney tissue, like all normal tissue, swells when it is bruised. The capsule surrounding the kidney is made of very tough fibrous tissue and limits the ability of the kidney to expand. Thus, when the tissue swells within this unyielding capsule it presses inward. The contrast between the wide, full spaces in the uninjured kidney and the narrow, compressed spaces in the contused kidney is usually very obvious and is the hallmark of this common injury.

As long as the capsule is not broken the kidney casts a distinct shadow on the x-ray film and its outline can be clearly seen. If the capsule is torn, blood from the damaged kidney tissue leaks out and surrounds the kidney, blurring this sharp outline. Again, the contrast with the shadow cast by the opposite uninjured kidney is usually striking.

Simple contusions and those accompanied by a tear in the kidney capsule heal without treatment. Many physicians recommend a fairly long period of bed rest or limited activity, but JP and I were never convinced that this was necessary. Traces of blood can be found in the urine for as long as three weeks, but as soon as the children are free of pain they usually can be allowed to do whatever they wish.

If the kidney is subjected to great force it may be ripped from the blood vessels that supply it or may be broken into two or more parts. Since Hypaque can only reach the kidney through its blood vessels, the infusion pyelogram following disruption of the blood supply shows no Hypaque at all on the injured side. Unless the torn blood vessels are repaired at once, the kidney cannot survive. Fortunately, these are rare injuries. Neither JP nor I ever saw one in time to save the kidney.

Nearly all of the children who require operation are those whose urine-collecting systems have been disrupted. The capsule and the kidney tissue are always severely damaged also, and usually the kidney has been broken into two pieces. If the break is near the center of the kidney, both halves may be sutured back together and the entire kidney saved. Often the lower pole of the kidney has been broken off and must be removed because it has been separated from its blood supply. In these children the torn collecting system in the main part of the kidney can be repaired with sutures and a major portion of the kidney saved. Usually this remaining portion is large enough to sustain good health should the opposite kidney be lost later in life.

The hallmark of this injury is the escape of urine containing Hypaque into the pool of blood that surrounds the kidney. The infusion pyelogram clearly shows the presence of opacified urine outside the kidney where no urine ought to be. This mixture of blood and urine is an ideal place for bacteria to multiply, and this accounted for the infections that caused some of the children whose records we reviewed to lose their kidneys. We have not seen a single such infection since we began to operate promptly on all children whose infusion pyelograms showed urine leaking through a tear in the collecting system.

As we continued to study children with injured kidneys we quickly discovered that the sooner after the injury we did the infusion pyelogram the better x-ray pictures we obtained. If we waited until the next day the damaged kidney tissue had sometimes become so swollen that there was little room for Hypaque in the compressed urine-collecting spaces. By doing the study within two to eight hours after the accident we were able to make the correct diagnosis and plan appropriate treatment in a very high percentage of cases without having to resort to more complicated diagnostic procedures.

We presented our findings to the hospital staff and it was agreed that all kidney injuries would be managed in the manner we recommended. About three years later JP and I summarized our results, comparing children treated before and after adoption of infusion pyelography and operations designed to conserve kidneys rather than remove them. We were surprised to find how much better our results had become.

I was invited to present our report to a joint meeting of APSA, the American Pediatric Surgical Association, and BAPS, the British Association of Pediatric Surgeons. The meeting was convened in Edinburgh, the home of our old friends Jimmie and Louie Mason-Brown. The president of BAPS opened the conference with a touching tribute to the lifework of this humble, gentle man. Louie was there, surrounded by a host of friends from both sides of the Atlantic, but Jimmie missed his big day. He died only a few weeks before we gathered to honor him.

31

Phoebe

While JP and I were gathering our data and working out the details of our report on kidney injuries a little girl with a different problem came to the hospital one Sunday morning and wormed her way deep into my heart. Bill and Tom were away, and I was making rounds, visiting each of their patients as well as my own, when the telephone operator paged me to come to the emergency room. I hurried down to find Dr. Baxter, our Chief of Staff, hovering anxiously over a stretcher on which a little four-year-old girl lay wrapped in sterile sheets. Sterile sheets like these were used only for burned children.

Beside Dr. Baxter stood his old friend, Dr. Reel, who before retiring had been Chief of Obstetrics at the medical school. Both men were deeply concerned, but Dr. Reel's concern was more than professional. This little girl was his granddaughter.

Phoebe had set her nightgown on fire while playing with a cigarette lighter. Her body had been severely burned, but her face, hands, and feet had been spared. She would have many deep scars, but just as clothing had caused the burn, clothing would hide most of the scars—if I could save her.

Dr. Reel's face reflected anguish not only because Phoebe was in pain and danger, but also because she would be cared for by a young stranger instead of by Bill or Tom whom he knew and respected. Dr. Baxter, as always, was very supportive of me, and assured his friend that I would do everything possible for his beloved grandchild. The old man grasped my hand, implored me to do my best, and left me to my work. As I lowered the sheets and saw the extent and depth of Phoebe's burn, I knew in my heart that my best would probably not be good enough. Only a miracle could save her.

I gave her some morphine and started an intravenous infusion. A team of residents arrived to help me, and together we cleaned the wound and applied a massive sterile dressing. As the morphine took effect Phoebe's pain diminished, and the anxious look on her face gave way to one of grim determination. This little girl was a fighter. Maybe, I thought, that would make the difference.

We took her to the burn unit where we gave her a tetanus booster and added penicillin to the fluid dripping into the vein in her arm. When we had made her as comfortable as possible, we gathered together in the nurse's station outside her room to go over our plan for her care. She would lose a tremendous amount of fluid into her burned tissue, fluid that we would have to replace minute by minute to prevent her from going into shock. Shock is not an emotional response, as is commonly believed, but a physical one resulting, in burned children, from loss of fluid from the blood. If recognized promptly, shock is usually easily corrected, but if not, it becomes irreversible and then is invariably fatal. Fortunately, I had been able to begin intravenous fluid replacement before shock had occurred, and with careful attention it should not now develop.

I reviewed the signs of inadequate fluid replacement so that everyone would be on the lookout for them. Among these are a rising pulse rate, a falling blood pressure, and a decrease in the hourly output of urine. Sometimes, even before these signs appear, children who are going into shock exhibit disorientation, talking to people who are not there, or giving unusual and unexpected answers to questions. They may seem to be in a twilight state between wakefulness and sleep, and when aroused by shaking or a loud command may become perfectly lucid again, deceiving the unwary.

At the opposite extreme is the danger of fluid overloading. When fluid runs into the vein too rapidly there are fewer signals to alert the doctor in time to avert catastrophe. The pulse and blood pressure do not change, but usually the urine becomes more copious and very dilute. With dramatic suddenness the capillaries in the lungs, millions of tiny blood vessels surrounding the air spaces, lose their ability to hold back the excess fluid in the blood. The air spaces become flooded, a condition known as pulmonary edema. If pulmonary edema is not treated rapidly and vigorously, the child dies from suffocation.

The first protection against either shock or pulmonary edema is an accurate assessment of the size and depth of the burn wound, allowing the doctor to determine how rapidly to begin fluid replacement. Dr. Chamberlain had taught me how to do this, and my assessment proved very accurate. Thereafter, constant vigilance is crucial to detect the earliest sign that the rate of replacement is too fast or too slow. It is small wonder that severely burned children have the best chance to survive if they are cared for in a well-organized burn unit where all the nurses and doctors are skilled in providing the demanding care they need.

There are many good burn units now, and most severely burned patients reach one within a few hours of injury. Such was not always the case. In fact, the very first burn unit in Ohio, for either children or adults, was established in the Columbus Children's Hospital by Tom Boles and John Terry at about the time Phoebe was born.

Phoebe's mother arrived just as we were finishing our conference at the nurse's station. I had never met Connie before, but I was to come to know her very well in the days and nights that lay ahead. She understood the gravity of Phoebe's situation, but never once did she let Phoebe know that she was worried. There was pitifully little that Connie could do for her little girl, but she needed desperately to be allowed to help. In addition to the natural urge to care for their children, mothers of burned children have a special need because deep down in their hearts they have a nagging feeling of guilt. If only Connie had been more attentive and alert, might she have prevented the terrible accident?

Covered by bulky dressings that prevented her from moving, Phoebe could not sit up to be hugged or comforted. Because of the ever-present danger of infection, Connie had to cover her familiar clothes with a sterile gown, her hair with a surgical cap,

and her face with a mask. She could not touch Phoebe or anything in Phoebe's room without wearing rubber gloves. None of
Phoebe's favorite toys could be brought to the hospital unless
they could be sterilized in a steam autoclave. Picture books turn
into soggy masses of pulp in an autoclave, and few dolls or
Teddy bears can withstand this brutal but necessary treatment.

Connie helped immensely just by being there where Phoebe
could see and hear her. After the first few days, during which
she was too sick to care, Phoebe loved to be read to. Connie sat
in the doorway of her room reading to her by the hour, fulfilling
in a small but important way her role as Phoebe's mother and
gradually assuaging the guilt she must have felt but never mentioned.

Word of Phoebe's trouble soon reached our home because
Phoebe's sister was in Peter's class in school. Every day when I
came home from the hospital Peter asked me about Phoebe. One
day he brought a message from the teacher asking if the children
could draw pictures for her. Provided they were big enough to
be seen from a distance we could hang them on the wall, but because of the danger of infection she would not be able to touch
them. Within a few days about thirty poster-sized pictures were
taped to the walls of Phoebe's room.

By the end of the second week I was beginning to feel more
optimistic about Phoebe's chances for recovery. She had responded to the early phases of our treatment, better than we had
any right to expect. Everyone who came near Phoebe loved her.
She was a dear little girl with a droll sense of humor, and was
very brave when we caused her pain, which we did each time we
changed her dressings. She did her best to respond when we
urged her to eat, but she needed far more in the way of nutrition
than she could take in without becoming nauseated. If pushed
too far, she simply vomited the food and fluid we forced upon
her. Despite our best efforts she rapidly lost weight, and every
day her little face became more drawn and pinched.

If Phoebe was to survive we would have to begin the long
process of covering her wound with skin grafts very soon. She
would need several grafting operations at weekly intervals, and
until her entire wound had been grafted she would not be out of
danger. Slowly, ever so slowly, the devitalized tissue came away,

leaving a healthy base on which we could begin to place the grafts.

I longed for some of the good old Debricin which we had found so helpful at Boston City Hospital before Castro cut off our supply.

Our daily dressing changes gave us only a piecemeal view of Phoebe's wound. We uncovered and redressed her chest before doing the same to first one arm and then the other. Then we turned her over and dressed her back. Finally we took her to the operating room, where after she was asleep we removed all the dressings at once. How huge the wound was! How thin and wasted Phoebe had become! We applied a small number of skin grafts to a portion of her back where her wound appeared ready to accept them. For the next few days Phoebe would have to lie continuously on her stomach.

There was a television set in Phoebe's room mounted high up on the wall opposite her bed. When she lay on her back she could see it well enough, but when she lay on her stomach she could not see it at all. The night after her operation I went to see her and was treated to a touching sight. Protruding from under Phoebe's bed were a pair of heavy workman's shoes. I crouched down to get a better look and found one of the hospital carpenters, wearing a sterile gown, cap, mask, and gloves, stretched out full length on his stomach on the floor beneath her bed. He was making final adjustments to a wedge-shaped structure he had made for her on his own time in the carpentry shop. When he was satisfied that he had it just right he placed a large mirror on it. By looking straight down toward the floor, Phoebe could see in the mirror the reflected image of the television screen.

For forty-eight hours we could not inspect the delicate grafts for fear of tearing them away with the bandages. As soon as I dared I gingerly lifted off a corner of the dressing. Not a single piece of grafted skin had begun to "take." The wound which had looked so pink and healthy in the operating room was covered with a dull gray film. Despite all of our careful precautions Phoebe's burn had become infected. Neither in Boston nor in Columbus had I ever seen a child survive when infection caused the first graft to fail. I tried to be optimistic, but I had to be truthful when Connie asked how the grafts were doing. I was utterly crushed and could not hide my deep concern.

As the days passed Phoebe grew desperately ill. Her temperature soared to 105 degrees, and she would eat nothing at all. She became drowsy and disoriented, not because she wasn't getting enough fluid, but because some of the millions of bacteria that were multiplying unchecked in her wound were swarming into her bloodstream. There was one last antibiotic to try. I had been hesitant to use it because it was known to be very toxic, but in the absence of any alternative I felt Phoebe's critical condition warranted using it. Having done everything I could for her, I stood in the doorway to say good night to her before going home to bed.

"See you in the morning, Phoebe," I said, not really expecting an answer. Phoebe muttered something unintelligible.

"What did you say?" I asked.

"I'll see *you* in the morning!" she replied, summoning up the old grit from somewhere within her. Before morning came Phoebe was dead.

How could I tell Peter? How do you talk about dying to a five-year-old boy? I needn't have worried. Like all little boys, Peter already knew many things his father hadn't told him.

"Did Phoebe die?" he asked simply.

"Yes, Peter, I'm afraid she did."

"Did you do something wrong?"

"No, I don't think I did, Peter."

"Well, where are all the pictures, in the wastebasket?"

Of all the children who have died under my care, losing Phoebe hurt me most. How I loved that brave and cheerful little girl! Had she sustained her burn today she almost certainly would have lived. Since that sad day in 1963 the care of burned patients has undergone tremendous improvement. In addition to the proliferation of organized burn units, a host of new medications have been introduced. Topical drugs that can be applied directly to the surface of the wound have done wonders to reduce the kind of invasive infection that cost Phoebe her life.

Skin grafts from other people still almost never "take" permanently, but these, as well as grafts from animals, offer invaluable temporary protection until strips of the patient's own unburned skin can be grafted. These strips of skin, only a few thousandths of an inch thick, can be passed through a device that cuts a series of uniform little slits in them so that the grafts can be stretched to resemble a lattice, covering many times the area they could cover without the slits. The diamond-shaped spaces in the lattice fill in as the skin grafts begin to take, and thus a large wound can be covered permanently in a single operation with skin taken from a small donor site.

Perhaps the greatest advance has been improved nutrition. Instead of the devastating starvation which used to be seen routinely, new techniques make it possible to prevent any weight loss at all, and this is at least as important in preventing infection as all of the dozens of new drugs.

Most important, had Phoebe been wearing non-flammable sleepwear, she would not have sustained the horrible burn at all. The federal regulation prohibiting the sale of flammable sleepwear has prevented countless tragedies like Phoebe's, and is one piece of government "interference" that must be kept in force.

32

We Go to Scotland

The invitation to speak in Edinburgh provided a nucleus around which Patty and I planned a family trip through Scotland, England, and Europe. It was the perfect time to take our children. Peter celebrated his eighth birthday on the boat on the way to Southampton. Amy was eleven, Kate fourteen, and Jeff sixteen. A year later Jeff might have been too old to put up with many of the activities that delighted his younger sisters and brother. A year or two earlier Peter would have been too young to keep up. As it was, we all had a wonderful time together, and I discovered many things about my children that I had been too busy or too preoccupied to learn before.

Believing that three weeks was too long to be away from the hospital, I stayed behind while Patty and the children went to England by boat. A week later I flew to London and picked up a rented car. The agent who met me at Heathrow airport obligingly drove me to the outskirts of London where I could learn on uncrowded highways how to drive on the left side of the road. I wondered how many Hertz employees would have done the same for a British subject arriving at Idlewild, as Kennedy airport was called in those days.

When we met at an old country inn the children were full of tales of adventures on the boat and at Stonehenge, which they had visited on the way up from Southampton. I had thought of Stonehenge as a place filled with mysteries that only an adult could comprehend, but this obviously had not been the case. I have always regretted not realizing how admirably the Children's Hospital would have functioned without me had I had the good sense to take the extra week off and go with them.

The British begin their theatrical performances an hour earlier than we do in America, a blessing for all, and doubly important if children are to enjoy them. Patty was sure the children would enjoy seeing a Shakespearian play performed by the world-famous company at Stratford on Avon. I was doubtful of their staying powers, but they remained glued to their seats through every word of *Timon of Athens*. I was surprised to find that Kate had studied *Timon* in school. I might have known this had I been more attentive at the dinner table at home, but I had no idea she knew more about the play than I did. Not only was she thoroughly familiar with it but she loved it, and as the play proceeded she took great delight in whispering messages in my ear about what would be happening next.

Having mastered in the Cotswolds the art of driving on the "wrong" side of the road, I drove us into the heart of Birmingham to take the train to Scotland. We had a few near misses, especially at "roundabouts," but we and the rented car arrived unscathed. Instead of having to find the rental agency, we were met at the railroad station by a uniformed employee who informed me as he collected the car that I had overpaid the agency some twelve pounds and a few shillings. Instead of giving me the expected form to fill out in triplicate, he reached in his pocket and refunded the full amount in cash. As I boarded the train I was full of warm feelings for the British.

It was a most comfortable train. Peter nestled snugly into his seat by the window and was soon fast asleep. The sun-drenched countryside through which we passed on the way to Scotland was about the only feature of the entire vacation that Peter missed.

After the opening session of the surgical meeting Louie Mason-Brown was free to show Patty and the children the sights of Edinburgh. One of the highlights of the city was the zoo, where dozens of penguins entertained their visitors. Patty adores penguins and has very fond memories of Edinburgh on their account. It rained most of the time, but the sun did come out one afternoon in time for me to join the family in a climb up the old tower, from which we had a panoramic view of the city. I remember the large patches of emerald-green grass that could be seen from this lofty perch.

It was fortunate that my talk was not scheduled on the first day of the meeting. If it had been, it would have been a disaster because I would not have known about the slide projector. In the United States, lantern slides come in two standard sizes. There are projectors for the large slides and other projectors for the small ones. In Europe, apparently, lantern slides came in several sizes and shapes, all of which the single ancient projector at the back of the auditorium in Edinburgh had been able to accommodate when it was new. With age it had developed a penchant for smashing the slides as it ejected them. In order to prevent the huge bulb from burning the slides, the projector had a cooling fan driven by a motor that made almost as much noise as a thrashing machine. The projectionist was an amiable and willing old retainer who unfortunately was nearly stone deaf. When a speaker wanted to call for his next slide he pressed a button that set off a buzzer in the back of the auditorium. Everyone in the audience could hear it, but the poor projectionist could not, and had to be poked by one of those near him before he would advance the slide. The talks given on that first day were unnerving experiences for even the most accomplished public speakers. I had visions of my carefully prepared lecture dissolving in a shambles.

Fidgeting uncomfortably in the seat next to mine was Mark Ravitch, who had advocated the use of barium enemas to reduce intussusceptions. I noticed in the program that he was scheduled to follow me on the podium the next day, and we resolved to team up to try to avert disaster. We rehearsed our talks together that evening and arranged a series of signals. Next morning Mark stood at the deaf old man's elbow, coaching him as to when to advance my slides and deftly catching them before they crashed to the floor on emerging from the noisy monster. I did the same for him, and both of our talks went off without a hitch, whereupon we relaxed and began to enjoy the proceedings. Apparently the British and European surgeons had had their share of problems in managing children with kidney injuries. Our use of infusion pyelograms and our suggestions as to ways of conserving kidney tissue when operations were necessary were well received and elicited a number of favorable comments.

Louie Mason-Brown invited us to lunch in her home, where we met her daughter and her son, who was part way through medical school. He was hoping to follow in his father's footsteps by becoming a surgeon. We were to see him a few years later in Columbus when he came for a period of surgical training under Dr. Zollinger. Louie proudly wore her spring suit, presumably made of a lighter tweed than her winter one. The spring tweed was nearly half an inch thick, just right for that sunny day in August.

From Edinburgh we drove down the coast and took the boat train to Copenhagen. Here there was another zoo with penguins, the Tivoli gardens, which are a paradise for children and adults, and the circus. We could have gone to the circus in Copenhagen every night for a week.

Though we had no guide in Copenhagen, Patty had been there before and knew what we all would enjoy. Having been to Elsinore Castle on her previous trip, she decided to send the children with me and do some shopping while we were gone. We set off with a driver who told me we would have time for one or two side trips along the way. I left the selection of these trips to him, and we soon found ourselves in line to buy tickets to the aquarium. Here were about fifty huge glass tanks containing fish from all parts of the world, some in salt water, some in fresh, some in warm water, and some in cold. Beside every tank was a map of the world with the area to which the fish in that particular tank were native outlined in red. I found this aquarium immensely interesting, but fifty tanks were too many for the children, and they were eager to pile into the car when we finally reached the exit.

The driver proceeded only a few miles before turning into the driveway of what appeared to be a large country estate. He got out of the car, lighted a cigarette and told us he thought we would enjoy this modern art museum. I remember looking at that cigarette and thinking that most of it would still be unsmoked when the children were done with a modern art museum. An hour later I had to drag Jeff away. His interest in art, which he later pursued to a fine arts degree in college, was first revealed to me that day on the way to Elsinore.

Elsinore is a fortress to delight the imagination of every boy and every man with a spark of boy left in him. From the parapets one can look across the water to the shoreline of Sweden, and it is easy to conjure up visions of glorious sea battles and of prisoners captured in desperate hand-to-hand combat being led off in chains to the gloomy dungeons. Kate and Amy, who are not warriors at heart, sat on the grass outside the castle watching with detached amusement as Peter explored nooks and crannies too small for me or Jeff to crawl into and periodically dashed back to headquarters to report what he had found.

After Copenhagen we went to Lucerne, the lovely little Swiss town at the end of a crystal-blue lake. We boarded a boat for a ride along the lake to the foot of Mount Riggi, which we ascended in a little cog-wheel train. We picnicked at the top in a field of wild flowers like the fields where Heidi used to play.

We spent a night in Amsterdam where the museum disappointed Jeff because it had no modern sculpture, and then returned to London. Here we stayed at the Hotel Connaught. Once in a lifetime everyone should stay at the Connaught. The dining room is a truly wondrous place, featuring, among other rarities, plover's eggs. We never tried any plover's eggs, but the reverence with which the waiter told us we could order them suggested that they must be among the world's greatest delicacies.

Tea at the Connaught was a sumptuous feast that served admirably as supper for the girls and Peter. They snuggled happily in their beds after tea, leaving Jeff free to go with us to the theater. He had been a good sport to adhere to the pace and whims of his younger sisters and little brother, but he greatly enjoyed a chance to do something without them. He carefully refrained from gorging himself on the sandwiches and pastries at tea time to save room for dinner with us after the theater.

We joined some friends whom Patty and the children had met on the boat and went together to see the crown jewels in the Tower of London and the changing of the guard at Buckingham Palace. We discovered that if we followed the horses home after the ceremony we could see their stable and pat them. The guards, so stiff and formal at other times, were very relaxed and friendly at the stable. Without their huge helmets they appeared to be scarcely out of their teens.

In Westminster Abbey, set in the stone floor, we saw the large tablet that is the British equivalent of our tomb of the unknown soldier. As we approached we found it surrounded by four German boys of about twenty years. One was haltingly translating the inscribed tribute to bravery for his companions who gazed respectfully upon it, perhaps oblivious, perhaps not, to the fact that the bravery of which they stood in solemn awe had been an all-out effort by the British to kill their fathers.

We sailed for home on the old *Queen Mary*, which the children found far less exciting than the *Niew Amsterdam* on which they had begun their voyage. Anticlimactic as this part of the trip might have been, it gave us time to review the sights we had seen and the things we had done together before we became immersed in our separate worlds in Columbus. We had looked at the same things, but we had looked through different eyes, and each of us had seen something the others had missed.

33

Kidney Transplants

When Dr. Zollinger agreed to let me come to Columbus and offered me a position in the Department of Surgery he asked me a penetrating question. "Anyone with your training can take care of patients," he said. "The question is, what else can you do?" I gave that nagging question a great deal of thought.

My practice was busy, varied, and interesting. I had plenty of patients to care for. In addition, I was becoming an effective teacher. Bill and Tom, whose experience was more extensive than mine, had more to offer the senior residents than I did, but I was more comfortable than they with junior residents and interns, and especially with medical students. Very few surgeons teach equally effectively at all levels. Just as some teachers are more at home teaching third graders than college students, some medical educators are more effective at laying an early foundation than at putting the finishing touches on doctors about to complete their training. Most doctors, looking back at their medical education, are hard pressed to name the phase that was most meaningful to them. In teaching, as well as in patient care, I was satisfied that I was making a useful contribution.

Research was equally important. Without research, teaching stagnates and patient care does not improve. The work JP and I had done with Tom Frye and Marc Rowe had been a respectable contribution to clinical research, but we had gone as far with kidney injuries as our imaginations would take us. It was time to look for something else.

In one of his more philosophical moments Dr. Child had talked to me about the promise of transplantation. The field was in its infancy, limited in almost every direction by the phenomenon of rejection. Corneas could be transplanted, permanently restoring sight to a significant number of people whose eyes were otherwise healthy. There are no blood vessels in the cornea of the eye. Virtually every other tissue is dependent upon blood vessels for survival. Not only do these blood vessels nourish the tissues, but they also carry to them whatever it is that causes the body to reject them. Only from one identical twin to another could organs like kidneys be transplanted with permanent success, but the results in identical twins were truly spectacular. It would not be very long, Dr. Child maintained, before some measure of control over the phenomenon of rejection would be achieved, and a young surgeon would do well to prepare himself for the day when kidney transplants between people other than identical twins became practical. Sure enough, not long after my training ended a few surgeons began to report more than an occasional success.

A prerequisite to kidney transplantation was an artificial kidney with which to prepare patients for the operation and upon which to fall back if the body began to reject the transplanted kidney. I would need an artificial kidney suitable for children. The available models were heavy and cumbersome. Even today, no artificial kidney is really portable, and none can be worn internally.

The world's first artificial kidney was invented in Holland by Dr. Willem Kolff. It was a very simple device consisting of a long tube of cellophane, flattened, wound in a coil, and immersed in a salt solution in a large tin can that originally had contained sliced pineapples. Blood from the patient circulated slowly along the inside of the cellophane tubing. Urea and other waste products in the blood made their way through tiny pores in the cellophane and were carried away with the fluid. The results of this dialysis, or "washing" of blood, were dramatic. Comatose patients slowly awoke and became ravenously hungry. They were restored for a brief time to reasonably good health, but as soon as the dialysis was terminated toxic wastes began to reaccumulate and they soon lapsed into coma again.

Several investigators in America developed artificial kidneys, each different in design, but all similar in that they exposed a thin film of blood to a salt solution separated from the blood by a sheet of cellophane. Some, like Dr. Kolff's original machine, were tubs containing a long coil of flattened cellophane tubing. Some held large sheets of cellophane between plastic boards with little grooves milled in their opposing surfaces. Dialysis with any of these machines was tedious and demanding, but without dialysis it was impossible to conceive of helping patients by transplanting healthy kidneys to them.

One of the devices available in 1965 caught my fancy. Developed in Buffalo by a Dr. MacNeil, it was attractive for several reasons. It was small, relatively simple to assemble, and it had a little pump to control the flow of blood that was said to be less damaging to blood cells than most of the other available pumps. The MacNeil dialyzer had the added advantage of coming from Buffalo, which was a short trip by air from Columbus. I could make several trips to Buffalo to learn to use it, and could quickly take it back for repairs if it broke down. I could go to Buffalo, or anywhere else, as often as I wished as long as I paid my own way.

Dr. Jim Allen had recently moved to Buffalo after completing his pediatric surgical training in Columbus. On my first trip he introduced me to the Anthone brothers, who were doing successful kidney transplants there. Although I could never be sure to which Dr. Anthone I was speaking, as they were identical twins, I found them both very friendly and informative. I told them I was exploring the possibility of doing kidney transplants in children, and they offered to help me in any way they could. Perhaps, they volunteered, I would like to see one of their patients.

I will never forget the man I met that day in Buffalo. He appeared in every way as healthy as I. He had come to the hospital only a few weeks before, pale, sick, and bloated with fluid that his failing kidneys could no longer eliminate. His mind was so clouded by the presence of accumulated waste products in his blood that he could only mumble incoherently. After a few treatments with Dr. MacNeil's dialyzer he had undergone a kidney transplant operation, and in less than a month had returned to work. One of the twins examined him briefly, drew a blood sample from his arm and measured his blood pressure, which was normal. He hurried back to his job, assuring me as he left that the Anthones were the greatest doctors in the world. It was easy to see why he thought so.

I flew back to Columbus, elated and inspired by what I had seen. Apparently my enthusiasm was contagious. JP had been very skeptical, but he soon agreed to help me. Bill, whose firm backing I would need, was fully supportive. Most important, the hospital administrator told me to proceed at full speed to order a MacNeil dialyzer for the Children's Hospital.

I flew back to Buffalo, placed the order, and watched carefully as Barbara Brown, the Anthones' nurse, assembled the machine and attached it to a patient. Then, under her watchful eye, I assembled a dialyzer myself. It was a slender stainless steel box resembling an elongated cigarette carton. At each end a small metal pipe protruded through the floor of the box, and over these pipes were fitted thin plastic plates about two inches square. Strips of flattened cellophane tubing extended the length of the box between these plastic plates. When fully assembled, there were about thirty strips of cellophane tubing lying one on top of another. If stretched end to end, the tubing would have been almost fifty feet long. Little grooves in the plastic plates were arranged in such a way that the blood traveled down one tube and back along the next, entering at the bottom and eventually emerging from the top. Another pair of pipes permitted a salt solution to circulate around and between the layers of tubing, accomplishing the same "washing" function as the salt water in Dr. Kolff's pineapple can. There were two little pumps, one for the patient's blood, the other for the dialyzing fluid. They were simple but rugged, and when assembled correctly after being dismantled for sterilization, were very dependable. A plastic container resembling a large wastebasket contained the reservoir of fluid. A small electric heater was immersed in the fluid to keep it at body temperature.

Each dialysis session lasted eight hours, preceded by about two hours of assembly and followed by at least an hour of dismantling and sterilization. Miss Brown did the whole job herself, with one of the Anthones in attendance for only a few minutes when she turned on the dialyzer. Miss Brown worked a very long day, but was so caught up in the excitement of what she was doing that she never was heard to complain.

To compensate for the quantity of blood contained in the dialyzer and the long tubes that connected it to the patient, a transfusion of blood from the blood bank was needed each time the dialyzer was used. The need for a pint of blood for every dialysis posed a number of problems. It was not unusual for a patient to require as many as thirty dialysis treatments before a suitable kidney donor could be found. Each bottle of blood had to be compatible with that of the patient. As the patient was exposed to the blood of many donors he gradually became sensitized to many subtle factors in donor blood, and finding compatible donors became more and more difficult.

In addition to the problems of matching blood to blood, there was the possibility that repeated transfusions might in some way sensitize the patient to substances in the transplanted kidney, enhancing the chance for rejection. At our early stage the question was largely academic, though very worrisome. We could not dialyze patients repeatedly without using considerable quantities of blood from the blood bank.

There was one more problem with donor blood. Fortunately, I discovered it in the laboratory before I dialyzed my first child. When our dialyzer arrived in Columbus I had to train a group of nurses to assemble and use it. After they had become proficient I scheduled several trial runs in the laboratory using dogs as "patients."

As anyone who has given blood knows, the bottle in which the blood is collected contains a small amount of fluid. In this fluid is a substance that combines with the calcium in the blood. With the calcium tightly bound, blood will not clot in the bottle or in the tubing leading to it. It regains its ability to clot when it mixes with the patient's blood, where it comes in contact with an abundance of calcium. The substance that binds the calcium is a different anticoagulant from heparin, which is used to prevent the patient's blood from clotting in the dialyzer. Blood containing heparin will not clot, no matter how much calcium is added to it.

On the morning of our first trial run I watched the nurse as-

semble the dialyzer and prime it by filling the cellophane tubing
with blood collected from a donor dog. We gave the "patient,"
who was sleeping peacefully under an anesthetic, a dose of
heparin. All was ready. I turned on the little pumps, and blood
and fluid began to circulate, just as I had seen them do in
Buffalo. The nurse had caught on very quickly. I turned to con-
gratulate her. Suddenly there was a loud pop, followed by a hiss-
ing noise like that made by an oscillating lawn sprinkler. The
tubing leading to the dialyzer had burst, spraying a stream of
blood over the walls and ceiling of the laboratory. The practice
run was over almost before it had begun. That was the morning
I learned that heparin must be added to the donor's blood as well
as given to the patient. As soon as I had turned the dialyzer on,
calcium in the dialyzing fluid had crossed the cellophane barrier,
and fifty feet of flat cellophane tubing had become plugged with
a solid blood clot. We spent the entire morning wiping up the
mess. Fortunately it was Sunday, and nobody was around to
enjoy the sheepish looks on our faces.

We called Barbara Brown and told her what had happened.
After she stopped laughing she apologized for not having told us.
She had forestalled any such disasters in Buffalo by having a
technician in the blood bank add heparin to the blood before
sending it down. No wonder I had not seen Barbara put it in.

After that messy incident we had only one more problem with
the dialyzer. Although I thought we had performed every step
of the assembly exactly as on previous occasions, this time the
dialysis fluid simply would not flow. After I had taken it apart
and reassembled it about ten times, I tucked the dialyzer under
my arm, drove to the airport and flew with it on my lap to
Buffalo. Barbara spotted the trouble at once. I had put in one little piece upside down. I blessed Dr. MacNeil for making the
components of his dialyzer so small and compact. About three
years later we abandoned his simple machine for a dialyzer that
used prepackaged cellophane tubing assembled and sterilized at
the factory. The new dialyzer saved us many hours, but when it
broke down I could not take it on my lap in an airplane. It was
as big and heavy as an upright piano.

34

Linden

It was not at all clear how many children would need kidney transplants, if and when I became competent to do them. A review of the autopsy records of the Children's Hospital suggested that in an average year two or three children died there of kidney failure. A relatively small fraction of them were infants, in whom the technical problems would be prohibitive, at least in the beginning. Perhaps two thirds of the rest might have been suitable candidates for kidney transplants. This wasn't very many. On the other hand, nobody knew how many children died of kidney failure elsewhere because their physicians, believing that we could do nothing for them, saw no useful purpose in sending them to our hospital. History had shown repeatedly that when a treatment for a previously incurable condition was found, patients with the condition appeared in unexpected numbers. I felt there was a distinct possibility that as many as ten or twelve children a year might be saved in Columbus if a sound kidney transplant program could be developed for them.

I would have to proceed step by step. The first step had been to purchase and learn to use an artificial kidney. Although one doctor and one nurse could easily do the work involved, it would be wrong to confine expertise in dialysis to me and one nurse because if one of us became ill our patients would be defenseless. It was easy to find nurses to train in dialysis. Finding a doctor was more difficult. JP had the interest but not nearly enough time. Bill and Tom were very busy, and especially so at the very times when they would be most needed—when I was not available. Providence came to my aid in the form of Arthur Pearson, a bright, energetic and devoted pediatric resident. Dr. Graham, who had replaced Dr. Baxter as Chief of Pediatrics, was very supportive, permitting the flexibility in Art's schedule that allowed him to participate. Art and I worked long hours together and became very close friends. We soon found that there are few endeavors that require more harmonious teamwork between physician and surgeon than managing children with advanced kidney failure.

After our initial tribulations with the dialyzer, our confidence in our ability to use it grew rapidly, and I realized that I should quickly become proficient in doing the transplant operation. The Anthone brothers were very willing to help me, and I went to Buffalo on two occasions to watch them perform the operation. On both days, after I had become air-borne en route to Buffalo, the operations had to be canceled.

One of the earliest pioneers in kidney transplantation was Dr. David Hume, Chairman of the Department of Surgery at the Medical College of Virginia. While a young resident at the Peter Bent Brigham Hospital in Boston, Dr. Hume had participated in the very first kidney transplant operations. Bill Clatworthy, who knew him, arranged for me to visit Dr. Hume in Richmond, and there I saw my first transplant operation.

The operation, although it must be done carefully, is basically very simple. A single artery supplies the kidney, and a single vein drains it. A single tube, the ureter, carries the urine to the bladder. Joining the artery and vein to counterparts in the patient and implanting the ureter into the wall of the bladder is all there is to it. The transplanted kidney soon becomes firmly seated in its new position and does not require any surgical maneuvers to fix it in place.

My first attempts in the dog lab were so crude that I was glad no one was watching, but with each practice session my technique improved. Suturing the little blood vessels was aided by a special needle holder designed for operations on the eye. It was a clever device which allowed the needle to be grasped and released with a minimum of jiggling, so that the needle would not tear the delicate vessels. One of the otolaryngologists lent me his operating microscope, which made the tiny needle look like a crowbar. The slightest motion or tremor was greatly magnified when seen through the powerful microscope, and at first I was able to use it for only short periods before becoming nauseated, an unexpected form of motion sickness. After a few days I was no longer troubled by this unpleasant sensation. Practice with the microscope is valuable during the learning phase, but after the required skill in joining small vessels has been acquired, it is not necessary to use a microscope during kidney transplant operations.

Before I had practiced the operation very often we used our dialyzer for the first time on a child. He was no stranger to any of us. Linden had come to the hospital as a newborn baby with a serious congenital malformation of his bladder. Bill had operated on him several times, fighting in essence a series of delaying actions as his kidney function progressively deteriorated.

Despite his many bouts of illness, Linden was invariably cheerful. His broad grin and sunny disposition endeared him to everyone. His physical growth was considerably retarded, though his mind was keen enough, and his wit, combined with his small stature, made him seem wise beyond his apparent years. He was actually ten years old, though he looked at first glance to be about seven.

During his tenth year Linden's stays in the hospital grew longer. He missed long stretches of school, and when he was able to go to his classes his advanced kidney disease made him so somnolent that he took in little of what he heard. Finally, just as we were becoming acquainted with our dialyzer, his kidneys failed altogether.

Neither JP, Art Pearson, nor I looked upon repeated dialysis as a satisfactory way of life for a child. Unless dialysis was being used to prepare children for kidney transplants that would free them from continued dependence on it, we felt we should not begin it at all. Within a few years dialysis would make it possible to maintain even small children in good health for many weeks, but even today dialysis is generally not a satisfactory permanent solution for kidney failure in children.

Still, we had to start somewhere. Linden's mother had died of kidney failure, and now his father saw Linden slipping away from him too. He willingly agreed to one dialysis treatment. Regardless of the outcome of this one attempt, Linden's father and I agreed the dialysis would not be repeated.

I made an incision in Linden's groin and inserted the large plastic tubes from the dializer into the main artery and vein in his leg. Though I used an injection of local anesthetic, I remember wondering if it was superfluous. Kidney failure had put Linden into a profound coma. I turned on the pumps and the dialysis was underway. I sent a specimen of Linden's blood to the lab. The BUN—short for blood urea nitrogen—in that initial blood sample was 180, ten times the normal value. The BUN provides a measure of only one of the waste products that accumulate when the kidneys fail to do their work, but it provides a handy guide to the effectiveness of dialysis. In four hours Linden's BUN had fallen from 180 to 85. Although this was still far above normal, Linden had been accustomed to functioning quite normally when his BUN was in this range. We had proved our point. Our dialyzer worked, and we knew how to use it. I turned off the pumps and prepared to remove the plastic tubes. As I did so, Linden sat up, opened his eyes and said, "Dr. Morse, I'm hungry!" He had returned from the brink of death in four short hours.

My hands shook as I removed the plastic tubes. It would be very hard not to repeat the amazing treatment, but it would not be fair to this gallant little boy. I wasn't ready to transplant a kidney to him, and I had given my word to his father that I would not toy with his life.

The waste products accumulated quickly again, and within forty-eight hours Linden had slipped peacefully back into his coma. By the time the next child came along, perhaps I would be ready to do a transplant operation. Linden's kidneys had failed too soon for me to help him, but in his final days he had served well the children who would come after him.

Late that night I received a disturbing phone call. Pete Sayers had been working for hours to save a little boy with a massive head injury. His condition was stable, he would live for several hours, but he would not recover. His parents, Pete said, were wondering if when he died I could use one of his kidneys for a transplant operation. I simply wasn't ready. Before I undertook such an operation I would need many hours of additional practice in the laboratory. Regretfully I hung up the phone and tried to go back to sleep. I stared up at the ceiling for what seemed an eternity. Memories of Linden, whom I had known so well, flashed through my troubled head. How brave he had been on the many occasions when I had drawn blood from his skinny little arm. How cheerfully he had accepted the news each time I told him that he had to come into the hospital instead of going home with his father. Over and over I heard him say, "Dr. Morse, I'm hungry." How sad it was that he soon would be leaving us.

I dozed fitfully until almost daybreak. I've often wondered whether I was awake or asleep when I finally said to myself, "Tom, you don't need all that practice! You're just scared! No one will blame you if you fail on your first attempt, but what if you succeed?"

I called the hospital. Pete's patient was still alive. His condition had not improved. He had only a few more hours to live. I had to try.

Linden's father drove a milk truck. He was already out in his truck, winding his way through the streets of Columbus. He wasn't expected back at the dairy until noon. It was to be one of the longest mornings I ever spent. A secretary at the dairy called several of his customers, but each time she called he had come and gone. She finally reached him and he called me at the hospital. I could promise him nothing, but he did not hesitate. "Go ahead," I heard him say, "and good luck to you and Linden!"

Early that evening death came to the little boy with the injured brain. JP, upon whom I had counted to remove the donor kidney, was away. There was nothing for it but to remove it myself.

To preserve the kidney while I was preparing Linden to receive it, I threaded a small tube into its artery and washed out the blood with ice-cold saline containing a little heparin. The warm kidney became almost as cold as a block of ice, and its deep red color was replaced by an ashen-pale pink.

I quickly located an artery and a vein in the lower part of Linden's abdomen. Clamping the vessels with little bulldog clamps, which are far gentler than their name implies, I divided them and sutured them to the artery and vein of the ice-cold kidney. With bated breath I released the clamps and watched the kidney's artery throb to the beat of Linden's heart. The kidney swelled, filling with warm blood, and became deep red again. I turned my attention to the ureter, and experienced the thrill of seeing a steady drip, drip, drip of urine flowing from it. By the time I had implanted the ureter and closed the long incision in Linden's abdomen he had passed nearly a pint of beautiful pale golden urine—more than his own kidneys had been able to make in nearly a month.

David Hume, whom I reached at his home in Richmond about midnight, gave us welcome advice as to how to prevent Linden from rejecting his new kidney. Two drugs were used, prednisone and Imuran. Prednisone, a drug closely related to cortisone, was quickly obtained from the hospital pharmacy, but no one had ever asked for Imuran before. There wasn't any Imuran in the hospital. There wasn't any in Columbus. A resident from Dr. Hume's service drove to the Richmond airport and put a small supply on a plane for us. Art Pearson met the plane, and we gave Linden his first dose of Imuran about six hours after his transplant operation ended.

Perhaps it was beginner's luck, but Linden got well enough to go back to school.

35

"You're on the News!"

News of Linden's transplant operation traveled throughout the hospital with the speed of lightning. Within twenty-four hours almost everyone—doctors, nurses, secretaries, and maintenance workers—knew that the kidney was working normally and that if rejection could be prevented, Linden had a chance for a new lease on life. Everyone who worked there considered Children's Hospital a special place, and even in the dullest of times I found their high morale an unmistakable and uplifting force. In the days that followed this spectacular event the feeling of pride and hope that pervaded the hospital was electric.

With so many people keyed up and excited it was truly remarkable that word of the event failed to reach anyone in the news media for a full week. In a sense it was a most newsworthy event, but in another sense Linden and his father were entitled to their privacy, and it was doubtless inevitable that their right to anonymity would clash with what newsmen referred to as "the people's right to know."

We were all overwhelmed, when the news finally leaked, by the intensity of the reporters' curiosity. Not satisfied with the story that a team of surgeons had operated successfully on a little boy, they demanded to know *what* surgeons had operated on *which* little boy. They vehemently reiterated their sincere conviction that newsmen, and newsmen alone, have the right to determine what is news.

With the help of the hospital's public relations officer we held a formal news conference at which I read a carefully prepared statement. It was by no means a first; it was only a first for Columbus. Dialysis was not new, transplantation was not new, the medications we were using to combat rejection were not new; they were only new to Columbus.

The principles governing resolution of conflicts between the right of the patient and his doctor to privacy and the rights of reporters to report had been carefully worked out and summarized in a document to which the Academy of Medicine and the leaders of the media had agreed. Evidently this document had gathered more than its share of dust. Never having done anything particularly newsworthy before, I was unaware of its existence. The newsmen and women, if indeed they knew of it, had conveniently forgotten about it. Despite our best efforts, the resulting publicity aroused a number of physicians in Columbus to anger, and more than one accused me, though never to my face, of glory seeking.

After a few days the furor died down, but not before Art Pearson had inadvertently admitted to a reporter that should the opportunity arise, I might well be able to use both kidneys of a future donor, transplanting one to each of two needy children.

Dr. Graham, as Chief of Staff of the hospital, was very concerned lest the media nightmare be repeated. At the same time he was very supportive of me, and thoroughly appreciated my difficult position. Dr. Zollinger, my ultimate boss in the Department of Surgery, was also concerned. Though he said not a word to me, he sent me a copy of the old document. As Dr. Graham and I read it, both for the first time, we were relieved to find that I and the hospital spokesman had, whether by instinct or accident, followed the terms of the agreement to the letter.

Dr. Graham arranged a meeting with representatives of the press, radio, and television. Again they were adamant that "the people have a right to know," and that only newsmen have the right to determine what is news. At the same time, they were sympathetic and clearly did not want to harm the hospital or its patients. They agreed to abide in the future by the provisions of the old agreement between the media and the Academy of Medicine, a job made easier for them by the fact that they felt these provisions were quite reasonable. We asked them if they felt the document should be revised, but they could come up with no suggestions for revision. Dr. Graham and I drove back to the hospital, satisfied that we had successfully resolved a difficult and potentially explosive problem.

The prednisone and Imuran, which we were giving with the long-distance help of Dr. Hume, were doing their job. Linden continued to produce copious quantities of normal urine, his temperature, blood pressure, and blood count remained in acceptable ranges, and his BUN soon fell to normal. The BUN doesn't tell the whole story as far as kidney function is concerned, since it measures only one of a number of waste products, but when the BUN is normal one can be pretty sure that the kidney is handling all aspects of its job in a reasonably normal fashion. Most convincing, Linden was flourishing. His puffy face and swollen feet resumed their normal appearance as his new kidney eliminated the water his old ones had retained. The weight that he now began to gain reflected his voracious appetite, and his strength and enthusiasm increased rapidly.

After the first two weeks we began to reduce the prednisone from the very high initial doses to a level he would be able to tolerate week after week. High doses of prednisone, especially when combined with Imuran, reduce the body's ability to ward off infection. At first we kept Linden in the same strict isolation we used for burned children, but after the dose of prednisone was lowered we allowed him to roam about the ward and mingle with other patients and their parents. His joyous response to his new freedom made us all aware of how oppressive solitary confinement is to children, especially to those who feel relatively healthy. We also could see something that I had not appreciated before. Much as he loved his father, who was both mother and father to him at home, Linden's life had been sadly empty after his mother died. More than any other little boy I knew, Linden evoked the mothering instinct in every nurse who looked after him.

Far sooner than I had expected, Art Pearson and and I had our second candidate for dialysis and transplantation. His name was Alvin. Though he had a chronic, long-standing kidney disease and had been in poor health for several years, the rapidity of his terminal kidney failure came as a surprise to the doctors who looked after him. He had been a patient of the Children's Hospital staff all his life, and Art knew him well, but unlike Linden, Alvin had never required surgery. I met him for the first time on the day his failing kidneys stopped making any urine at all.

We knew that the chances of finding a donor for Alvin within a few days were remote, but encouraged by Linden's progress, we decided to embark on a series of thrice-weekly dialyses, hoping that we could sustain him until a suitable donor appeared. We had no idea how long this would be.

Alvin responded as dramatically as Linden to his first dialysis, and thereafter improved steadily, though not nearly as rapidly as Linden had after his transplant operation. It was clear that dialysis was a superb crutch upon which to lean until a transplant could be performed, but it fell far short of the ideal definitive treatment of kidney failure in children.

Late one afternoon a little girl was brought to the emergency room in critical condition. She had bounded out of a school bus in front of her home and had run into the path of an oncoming truck. Her father and mother followed on the heels of the ambulance and waited for three hours as a team of doctors and nurses struggled to save their little girl. Every wound could be repaired save the one to her head. Provided the respirator continued to breathe for her, she might live in a coma for as long as a week, but her brain was dead, and recovery could not be hoped for.

Having watched the efforts of the emergency room staff, the parents were convinced that nothing that might have been done to save their daughter had been omitted. When Art Pearson told them the encephalogram proved that her brain was dead they believed him, and they willingly gave us permission to transplant one of her kidneys. At least some good could come to someone from this unexpected and devastating tragedy.

This time JP was there to help me. As I opened Alvin's abdomen and prepared the vessels to which I would suture the artery and vein, JP removed one of the little girl's kidneys and ran the cooling solution through it. Before putting Alvin to sleep the anesthetist had happened to glance in the operating room where JP was working and received such a shock that he was not sure he could go through with his part of the procedure. The little girl had lived next door to him and was his own daughter's best friend.

Art Pearson, who was involved in every phase of Alvin's care except the operation itself, paced nervously up and down outside the operating room. As the cold, pale kidney was carried through the door from JP's operating room to mine, the anesthetist called out the time. It was exactly eleven o'clock.

Two minutes later Art poked his head through the door and in a mournful voice reported, "You're on the eleven o'clock news!" The operation was still in progress. How could the news have leaked? What had happened to our agreement with the media?

Dr. Graham and I had plugged all the holes except one. In my excitement I had failed to ask the little girl's father the one key question, "What do you do for a living?" He had signed the consent forms, phoned his boss to tell him what had happened, and taken his sorrowing wife home to their strangely empty house.

His boss ran a television station.

36

Rhonda

The immunologic matches between Linden and Alvin and the unfortunate little strangers who gave them their kidneys must have been very close. We were incredibly lucky that neither kidney was rapidly rejected. Prednisone and Imuran could overcome the body's attempts at rejection if the match were sufficiently close, but even the kidneys of brothers, sisters, fathers, and mothers were often rejected. As Dr. Hume observed, "The surprising thing is not that the drugs don't always work, but that they ever work at all."

The only indicator we had that our donors and recipients might be compatible was that they had the same blood types. This is essential, but there is far more to the phenomenon of rejection than can be measured by matching red blood cells. Tissue typing, comparable to blood typing but more complicated, was in its infancy. The tests required many hours and were done in only a few laboratories throughout the country.

If a patient were fortunate enough to have a number of close relatives willing and able to give him one of their kidneys, tissue typing might help to select the one whose kidney was least likely to be rejected. Living donors who were not related to the patient were used infrequently because the failure rate was so high. Many altruistic people were willing to request in their wills that their kidneys be transplanted when they died, but time and logistics nearly always precluded carrying out their wishes. Most donors other than close relatives were accident victims whose brains had been injured beyond all hope of recovery but whose hearts were still beating when they arrived at the hospital. For these donors tissue typing was usually out of the question because there wasn't time to do it.

The ethical considerations involved in declaring a patient dead while his heart was still beating received very concerned attention. Parents and relatives found acceptance of death under these circumstances particularly difficult, despite all the careful precautions that were taken to prevent unfortunate decisions.

The interests of the injured child and those of the patient waiting to receive a life-saving kidney were clearly at odds. To participate in caring for both of them would be to place oneself in an ethically untenable position. We carefully insisted that separate teams of doctors and nurses be responsible for their care.

The most reliable single criterion of brain death was a "flat" electroencephalogram. The electroencephalograph measures the brain's electrical activity. Little pens in the machine record on a moving strip of paper a series of wavy lines punctuated by rhythmically spaced high peaks and deep valleys. In the absence of electrical activity there are no "brain waves." The electroencephalograph records a straight, or "flat" line. Recovery after a "flat" electroencephalogram is very, very rare, but it has been known to happen. At least two "flat" encephalograms recorded several hours apart are required. The ultimate responsibility for declaring that the donors had no hope for recovery was mine, and in every instance I am satisfied that my decisions were proper.

Just as a cardiac surgeon cannot function effectively without the help of a cardiologist, it was clear that our transplant program could not flourish without a nephrologist, a pediatrician skilled in the medical care of children with advanced kidney diseases. Despite his limited experience, Art Pearson had served us well in this role, but Art was a resident in training and had only a few more months in which to complete all the requirements of a pediatric residency. Thereafter he would have to fulfill a military commitment. It was my hope that after he had satisfied this obligation he would go on to receive additional training in pedi-

atric renal diseases and join the staff as a fully qualified nephrologist. This would require an absence of at least three years.

The fact that we had a dialyzer and the rudiments of a kidney
transplant program made the position of nephrologist at Children's Hospital particularly attractive, and Dr. Graham succeeded in persuading Dr. Carl Nelsen to join the staff. Carl
proved a most valuable addition, not only to my transplant patients, but also to hundreds of children with less serious kidney
disorders. He had unlimited enthusiasm and a tremendous capacity for work. Word of his expertise spread rapidly, and in a very
short time the number of children coming to the hospital with
kidney problems more than doubled. Art Pearson did not feel
threatened. By the time he could return there would be plenty of
work for both of them.

Carl was in full agreement that endlessly repeated dialysis was
not satisfactory treatment for children whose kidneys had permanently failed. For them transplantation, with all its risks and
problems, was preferable. There were, however, some children
with short-term kidney failure for whom dialysis could provide
temporary support while their kidneys recovered. In addition, a
few types of poisons could be removed with dialysis, often
speeding recovery and occasionally saving a life. Carl, Art, and I
worked closely together whenever dialysis was used and enjoyed
a number of successes with it.

Considering the odds, it was inevitable that one of our transplant operations should end in failure. Little did we suspect, JP,
Art, and I, when Carl introduced us to Rhonda, how much she
would come to mean to us, or how tightly she would draw us
together in an effort to help her get well. It would take more
than one failure to defeat Rhonda.

Although she was six years old, Rhonda weighed only thirty-
two pounds. She was a petite and utterly feminine charmer, naturally blonde and even more fair because she was anemic. Her
hair was thin and brittle, lacking the luster it once had when she
was healthy. Only her eyes were untarnished by the dulling
effect of waste products her kidneys could no longer eliminate.
Those blue eyes, that followed us everywhere, seemed to remind
us, "I am open and honest with you. You be open and honest
with me." We always were.

Carl had skillfully supported Rhonda for many weeks, delaying as long as possible the inevitable moment when her failing kidneys would completely cease to function. This he did by giving her a monotonous diet containing only minute amounts of waste products for her kidneys to eliminate. Since her kidneys had a limited capacity for work, the object was to restrict in every possible way the amount of work they were called upon to do. Even water was allowed in only very small amounts, but Rhonda cheerfully ate the tasteless food and put up with her constant, nagging thirst.

Despite these strict measures the day finally came when her little kidneys could no longer make even a few drops of urine. Carl asked me to place a Scribner shunt in her arm so she could be dialyzed while we waited for a kidney donor. It was a simple device that permitted using the same artery and vein for dialysis over and over again. Without this ability, especially in small children, the number of dialyses one could hope to perform would have been severely limited. Like many medical advances, the Scribner shunt has had its day and now is rarely used.

The shunt consisted of bits of flexible Silastic tubing and stiff tapered tips made of Teflon. The Silastic resembled very soft rubber in that it could be molded to any desired shape, from which it could be stretched or bent but to which it sprang back when released. It differed from rubber in being transparent and in having a smooth, "unwettable" surface to which blood could not cling and begin to clot. The Teflon tips, about an inch long, were rigid and broke when one attempted to bend them, but they had the same "non-wettable" property that discouraged blood from clotting.

The tapered Teflon tips could be inserted into blood vessels, holding them wide open even when surrounded by a tightly tied ligature of silk. The hubs of these Teflon tips were seated in the ends of Silastic tubes that were led out through the skin and joined together with a short Teflon connector. Blood, propelled by the beat of the patient's heart, emerged through the skin via the soft Silastic tubing and returned to enter the vein. As long as the blood was kept moving, it had little tendency to clot, and many Scribner shunts could be kept in place for a month or more. Whenever dialysis was needed, the Silastic tubing was

gently clamped, the Teflon connector removed and the ends of
the shunt connected to the long tubes leading to the dialyzer.
Heparin was needed to prevent clotting only during dialysis sessions.

The Scribner shunts were a godsend for little patients like
Rhonda, but they had to be handled with extreme care. Only
two silk threads anchored the tips in place, and the danger of
dislodging the shunt was constantly present. Between dialyses the
shunt had to be bandaged securely in such a way that the doctor
could easily remove the dressing but the child could not. Even
the most tractable and understanding children have insatiably curious fingers. An alert nurse found Rhonda drifting off to sleep
one night, her arm in a rapidly widening pool of blood. Had the
dislodged connector not been quickly replaced she would have
bled to death through the very device that had been placed in
her arm to save her life.

Transplant operations involving fatally injured donors were always performed under emergency conditions, usually it seemed,
in the middle of the night. Rhonda's was no exception. We did
everything we could to minimize delay. As always, an operating
room was ready and waiting, with instruments and drapes sterilized ahead of time. Saline containing heparin, with which to
flush out and cool the donor's kidney, was kept in a refrigerator
held constantly at a few degrees above the freezing point. JP and
I were close to our phones and could arrive in the operating
room in a very short time. Nevertheless, the kidney I transplanted to Rhonda that night did not produce a single drop of
urine, presumably because we had not been able to act quickly
enough.

There was a chance, if dialysis were repeated at regular intervals, that after a week or two the kidney might begin to function, but it never did. After giving it every opportunity I sadly
removed it, and we went on as before, supporting her with our
artificial kidney while we waited for a second chance. Far from
discouraged, Rhonda accepted this disaster as a temporary set-
back. She wanted to live, and was serenely confident we would
see to it that she did. None of us shared her confidence, but we
could not come near her without renewing our determination to
try.

We went on all summer, dialyzing Rhonda three times a week, trapped in a commitment from which none of us ever considered backing away. Two possible donors appeared in our emergency room, but neither could be used because they did not have Rhonda's blood type. One after another, four Scribner shunts became gradually plugged with blood clots and had to be removed. I had to place the fifth in her leg because there were no suitable vessels left in either arm. No one admitted it, but we all knew we were running out of time.

Art Pearson finally gave voice to the obvious conclusion that had secretly haunted each of us. We should give Rhonda one of her mother's kidneys before it was too late. Considering our limited experience it seemed scarcely justifiable to take such a risk. Hadn't we had more than our share of good fortune with Linden and Alvin? Rhonda's mother seemed healthy enough, but how could we be sure that removing one of her kidneys might not endanger her health or shorten her life? Rhonda was a tiny little girl. Wouldn't her mother's kidney be too big for her? We had failed with her once already. It would be tragic to fail again and lose one of her mother's kidneys in the effort.

Rhonda's mother had more than her own wishes to consider. Even if she wanted to go through with the operation, would it be fair to her husband and her son to risk her life? After careful discussion the family decided it would. If she could pass all the tests she would be ready when we were.

We had never screened a potential living donor before, but on checking with Dr. Hume and the Anthone brothers we found that the procedure had become pretty well standardized. An internist took a careful medical history and performed a thorough physical examination. He found her perfectly healthy. A battery of blood and urine tests were normal. An intravenous pyelogram showed two normal kidneys. So far there was no contraindication to proceeding. We had to wait several days for the results of tissue typing tests, and when these finally came they showed a class "B" match between Rhonda and her mother, not the best, but acceptable. There was one more hurdle, an arteriogram which would show us the anatomy of the blood vessels supplying the kidney we proposed to transplant. We had saved the arteriogram until last because it carried a slight risk to Rhonda's mother, a risk she would not have to take had any of the other tests disqualified her.

We took her to the X-ray Department. Tom Frye slipped a long slender tube into her aorta and injected a bolus of radiopaque material at the point from which the arteries to her kidneys were expected to arise. She looked huge, lying on the x-ray table where we were accustomed to seeing babies and little children.

The x-ray machine made a thunderous clatter as more than a dozen films were exposed in rapid succession. The early films showed a beautiful artery, large and straight, leading to each kidney. The films exposed a few seconds later showed the renal veins, more faintly outlined because the opaque material had been diluted with blood in its passage through the kidneys.

At first glance, everything looked normal, but when we studied the films carefully we could see a second artery, much smaller than the main one, leading to the upper pole of each kidney. It was not unusual for a kidney to have two arteries, though one was the rule. Had only one of the kidneys had an extra artery we would have left it in place and transplanted the other, but we did not have that choice. Either we must abandon the thought of using Rhonda's mother as a donor or we must deal somehow with this second artery. When one attempted to suture so small an artery a clot usually formed on the suture line and occluded the vessel. Perhaps it didn't matter. Perhaps we could just tie off the little artery and forget it, depending on the main artery to nourish the entire kidney. If too much kidney tissue were dependent on that little artery the kidney would suffer an infarct, as does the muscle of the heart when a small branch of a coronary artery becomes occluded. If the infarct were small, it would heal, leaving an insignificant scar, and the kidney would function as if nothing had happened. If the infarct were larger, and particularly if it were to become infected, the whole kidney might be lost.

JP consulted at length with a colleague at the Cleveland Clinic who advised him to tie off the vessel. He had done this on two occasions, he said, and neither patient had suffered any ill effect.

Our tissue match was not perfect, our kidney's anatomy was

not perfect, and our experience with living donors was nil, but we decided to go ahead. Once Rhonda's operation was underway it would take me about twenty minutes to expose the site for the kidney to lie in and prepare the vessels to which I would attach it. JP, working in an adjacent operating room, would need nearly two and a half hours to remove the kidney. Rhonda's mother was a big, muscular adult; Rhonda was a scrawny little mite. I gave JP a two-hour head start.

Carl and Art sat with me in the surgeon's lounge, watching the hands of the clock crawl around the dial, and I shared with them the frustrating inactivity that Art had endured alone while I was operating on Linden and Alvin. He made no effort to conceal his enjoyment at watching me fidget and squirm. When a nurse told me my operating room was ready at last, I felt like a hockey player released from the penalty box. Poor Carl and Art, not being surgeons, had nothing to do but continue to wait.

Our timing had been nearly perfect. I was ready and waiting, with only a few minutes to spare, when the ice-cold kidney arrived from the operating room next door. It looked huge as I placed it in its new location, low down in Rhonda's right side, but there was plenty of room for it. JP had selected the mother's left kidney because its vein was longer than the vein on the right. Now it lay reversed from its original orientation, the back of the kidney toward the front and the upper pole at the bottom, to facilitate suturing the vessels together. Kidneys work equally well upside down.

Most of the kidney was very pale pink, the result of JP's flushing it with ice-cold saline. The upper pole, now at the lower end, was not nearly so pale. That was the part supplied by the little artery that JP had tied off. The ice-cold saline had not reached it. After the operation Rhonda's blood would not reach it either. This portion would die and be replaced by a scar. It was only a small bit of tissue, perhaps 10 percent of the kidney, but it looked ominously large as I began to suture the vessels. When this had been done and the clamps removed, Rhonda's pulse accelerated as her heart took on the added burden of perfusing the big kidney. In a few minutes it settled to its new task, and the pulse slowed to a normal rate. The kidney became warm and red as it filled with Rhonda's blood and began at once to produce pale golden urine, the first drops of urine Rhonda had made in more than four months.

JP's operation and mine, which had begun two hours apart, ended at almost exactly the same moment, and we gathered with Carl and Art in the surgeon's lounge for coffee. The finest champagne could not have tasted better than the coffee in those four Styrofoam cups. Luck was with us, more luck than we had any right to expect.

37

Rejection?

With the transplanted kidney functioning normally our chief concern was that Rhonda's body would try to reject it. Occasionally rejection came on with a rush and quickly overwhelmed any attempt to stop it, but usually it was a more indolent process, giving us at least a little time to apply the few available preventive measures.

The early warning signs included a rising temperature, a rising white blood cell count, and tenderness in the area surrounding the transplanted kidney. These were non-specific signs, typical of inflammation, and could be caused by infection as well as rejection. They could also be caused by a small leak of urine from the point at which the transplanted ureter was sutured to the bladder. The other indicators, a rising blood urea nitrogen and a decreasing urine output were more specific, suggesting that rejection was interfering with the kidney's ability to do its work. Even these indicators could have other causes, such as obstruction of the ureter or a clot forming on the sutures joining the vessels together. Usually when the problems were of a mechanical nature the signs of inflammation were absent, but when fever, elevation of the white blood count, and tenderness were accompanied by signs of deteriorating kidney function, rejection, rather than a surgically correctable condition, was nearly always responsible.

Combating rejection was based on two premises. The first was that every patient except an identical twin would try to reject a transplanted kidney. The second was that the attempt at rejection would be most intense in the first few weeks after transplantation. Prednisone and Imuran were given to every patient from the moment the operation was completed. After the first few days the initially high dose of prednisone could usually be gradually reduced as the threat of rejection diminished. This threat would never disappear completely, and the drugs would be continued as long as the transplanted kidney continued to function, hopefully for the rest of the patient's life.

The dose of Imuran was usually kept constant. The maximum dose was related to the body weight. At thirty-two pounds, Rhonda tolerated about one-fifth the amount generally used for adults. Too much Imuran drastically reduced the number of white blood cells in the blood, removing a vitally important protection against infection. As long as the white blood count remained in the normal range Imuran seemed to have few adverse effects, at least in the early months. No one knew for sure what the long-term effects of giving Imuran to little children might be.

Prednisone, like all medications related to cortisone, had many undesirable side effects. Primarily, it interfered with the body's ability to combat infection. For this reason alone, it was imperative to give it in the lowest dose that would suppress rejection. It retarded growth, an unimportant effect for adults, but harmful to little children. In high doses it interfered with the menstrual cycle or abolished it altogether. This would be of little immediate consequence to Rhonda, but might be a problem later. Finally, it caused profound cosmetic changes. The skin of the abdomen developed unsightly streaks similar to those seen in some women who have borne several children. It also gave rise to an accumulation of fat about the shoulders, aptly described as a "buffalo hump," and imparted to the face an unattractive round, puffy configuration known as a "moon face." These cosmetic changes were unimportant in a physical sense but were critically important psychologically. They often prompted teenagers to discontinue taking the drugs, usually without telling either their parents or their doctor. Giving enough prednisone to hold rejection in check while minimizing its many side effects was a complicated business.

Because rejection typically was most likely to occur in the early weeks we began with the maximum dose of Imuran and a relatively high dose of prednisone. If rejection threatened, the prednisone could be increased temporarily but the Imuran could not. If increasing the prednisone did not halt rejection a small dose of x-ray irradiation could be administered to the kidney. If these measures failed, there was nothing to do but accept defeat, remove the kidney and return to dialysis, hoping to find a new kidney with a closer immunologic match—if we still had a living patient. In the years following Rhonda's transplant operations survival of patients has improved considerably, partly through better methods of suppressing rejection, but also from improvements in managing patients whose transplanted kidneys have been rejected.

For the first few days Rhonda's recovery seemed almost too good to be true. By the time her mother was able to get out of bed and visit her, she was bright and cheerful, virtually free of discomfort, and eating everything in sight. We knew she had been sick, but as so often happens when a long-standing condition is suddenly corrected, we could only appreciate in retrospect how far below normal she had fallen. Each of us had witnessed gratifying recoveries, but few had filled us with such joyous exhilaration.

The second week was a nightmare. Rhonda suddenly lost interest in food. Her temperature rose a degree or two. Her white blood count, which had been pushed to the lower limit of normal by the combined effects of Imuran and prednisone, gradually rose despite continuance of the drugs. The area of her abdomen surrounding the transplanted kidney became tender, but more worrisome was the fact that her entire abdomen began to swell. Her urine output fell to a fraction of its previous rate, and her BUN, which had fallen to normal, rose an average of fifteen points a day. We doubled the dose of prednisone without effect, and doubled it again. An x-ray of her abdomen showed a diffuse, cloudy haze; the swelling was caused by the rapid accumulation of fluid. None of us had heard of this as a complication of rejection.

JP suggested that all of these sinister findings could be explained by a large leak of urine. Possibly the sutures joining the ureter to the bladder had given way. Perhaps the kidney was working normally but the urine, instead of flowing directly to the bladder, was leaking into her abdomen. If we could prove it, perhaps I could repair the leak. We placed a small catheter into her bladder and filled it with Hypaque, hoping that some of the contrast material would leak out and prove JP correct. Surgeons don't usually welcome evidence that their operation has gone awry, but this was one time when I devoutly hoped it had. The x-ray was completely normal. This did not prove conclusively that my suture line was intact, but I felt it was pretty strong evidence. If Rhonda was rejecting her kidney, the last thing she needed was an operation to repair something that did not need repairing.

Kidneys that are not working do not excrete Hypaque when one attempts to obtain an infusion pyelogram. Perhaps there was still enough kidney function to give an acceptable series of x-rays. I injected the Hypaque and saline for an infusion pyelogram. On the x-ray film I was amazed to see a heavy concentration of Hypaque within the kidney. Even more amazing was the fact that the entire abdomen was more hazy than it had appeared on a film exposed only minutes earlier. The ureter wasn't leaking; the *kidney* was leaking! The infarct caused by tying off the little artery had extended to the collecting space in the center of the kidney.

Dealing with the infarct turned out to be incredibly simple. In the operating room I made a minute incision over the lower pole of the kidney, and from this little incision gushed four or five quarts of clear, golden urine. Merely placing a drain through the abdominal wall to the kidney allowed the tissues to collapse around it, sealing the leak and permitting the infarct to heal. When the drain was withdrawn about a week later the opening closed of its own accord, and all of the urine traveled to the bladder as it was supposed to. The BUN had not risen because of rejection. The kidney had excreted urea normally into the urine which had then made its way to the abdomen where the urea was reabsorbed into the blood.

For more than ten years her mother's kidney supported

Rhonda without a serious threat of rejection. The scrawny little mite grew into a vivacious teenager, requiring so little prednisone that she never was threatened by infection. She was affected by the drug, however. When she graduated from high school she was barely five feet tall, and her face, though exquisitely beautiful to those of us who looked after her, was rounder and fuller than it would have been without prednisone.

She came to the hospital infrequently after the first few years. There seemed no reason to make her come more often, as her tests were always normal. Except for one overnight stay in the hospital each year, for tests that were difficult to do in an office, I saw her briefly every four to six months. Carl left the hospital to accept another position. Art Pearson did not return after his military service. JP received regular reports from me, but rarely saw her himself. Preventing rejection was up to me. Lulled by her long unruffled course, I fell asleep at the switch, forgetting a lesson I should have remembered from my days at Bellevue. All teenagers rebel at some time against taking medicine day after day. Diabetic teenagers rebel against giving themselves daily injections of insulin, and often make themselves gravely ill before they accept their continuing need for it. Why should Rhonda be different?

One day Rhonda looked at herself in the mirror and decided she didn't like what she saw. Without telling a soul she abruptly stopped taking her medicines. Nothing catastrophic happened, and she went cheerfully on her way, unaware that rejection was silently beginning to do its deadly work. The decline was so gradual that she was able to ignore it until her kidney was utterly destroyed. When she finally came to the hospital she was once more on the threshold of death.

It was too late for her four old friends to help her. Shortly after her first transplant Dr. Jim Cerilli had joined our surgical department. Jim was a thoroughly trained transplant surgeon. JP and I were amateurs. We had identified a need and briefly filled it, but it was time to turn transplantation over to an expert. We stopped doing transplants, satisfied that he could do them better. Under his leadership Ohio State University developed a fine transplant record, and Jim has become recognized as a leader in the field.

Jim put Rhonda on dialysis, removed the rejected kidney, and eventually gave her a third transplant. Having learned a bitter lesson, Rhonda now takes her medicine regularly. Three months from this writing she will graduate from nursing school.

She wants to work at Children's Hospital.

38
Storm Clouds

We felt an irresistible urge to move to the country. Patty was intrigued with the idea of building a house, whereas I leaned toward remodeling an old one. We had even gone so far as to tramp around the countryside, looking at possible building sites, when the ideal compromise fell into our laps. We were able to buy fifteen acres of beautiful land surrounded on three sides by woods in which there were miles of trails for hiking and riding. One of these trails wound its way through a grove of huge beech trees, said to be the only stand left in Ohio that had never been cut.

The former owner had acquired the land just before the Korean War, which, like the Second World War, had caused shortages of building materials. Having selected the site on which he proposed to build the house of his dreams, he constructed a smaller but very functional one on a secondary site and bided his time. Some eight years later, when building restrictions eased, he built the second house overlooking a pond which he stocked with blue-gills and bass.

The place would not have been satisfactory for us when the children were little, as each house had only two bedrooms, but now that they were older, with Jeff and Kate away at college most of the time, the arrangement was ideal. We lived very comfortably for a time in the little house while we made a series of changes in the bigger one. Chuck Frank, who was both architect and builder, did beautiful work for us, completely remodeling the kitchen and adding a new living room with beams in the ceiling and a cozy fireplace. There was a screened porch overlooking the pond. It was delightful in summer but useless in winter until we enclosed it with large windows that preserved its openness but made it warm on even the coldest days. It was our introduction to the possibilities of passive solar heating. With the addition of a third bedroom, complete with abundant closet space, our home became the envy of our formerly skeptical friends and made life in the country a joy that we appreciated all the more for having lived in the city so long.

Near the original house was a small building that served as a tool shed and stable for an ancient horse who could enter at will from a three-acre pasture. The mild winters made it possible for the horse to be out nearly every day of the year, greatly reducing the work of caring for her.

The ancient horse left with the former owner, but was soon replaced by Davey, a sturdy Morgan gelding raised by my father and mother. Davey had had a successful career in the show ring but had not been trained to jump. All the trails had jumps over which my riding companions sailed easily on their big hunters. Davey instinctively knew how to jump, but how and where he would land was always a question, and he did not seem to enjoy jumping very much. There was a way around every jump, so Davey and I had no trouble keeping up with the others. He loved the company of other horses, bucking enthusiastically whenever we met them on the trail. Sam, our exuberant black Labrador, went everywhere with us, and usually, though not always, returned when we did. Davey had an uncanny ability to see in the dark, which greatly extended my opportunities to ride, as dusk was often approaching when I came home from the hospital.

After a year Davey was joined by Gracie, and his life was complete. The two of them grazed side by side in the pasture, never more than a few feet apart, and huddled together in the stable when it rained or snowed. Davey would have been dismayed to learn that his beloved Gracie was his half sister.

Gracie had characteristics that discouraged Patty from riding her. She had little enthusiasm for getting her hooves wet, and enjoyed brushing close to the trees on the edge of the trail. Saplings yielded when a rider's knee crashed against them, but the huge beeches were unforgiving. In the dark Gracie behaved as if she were as blind as a bat. Her chief virtue, in addition to her role as Davey's adored companion, was that she apparently did not taste very good. There was a long season every summer when the flies persecuted Davey unmercifully. During the hot weeks Gracie, whom the flies avoided as if she had arsenic in her veins, was more fun to ride despite her idiosyncracies.

Moving to the country was hard for Amy at first. She had lived all her life in a city or suburb, and was appalled at the prospect of being so far from her friends. Fortunately, the move coincided with her sixteenth birthday, and a driver's license did wonders to ease the pain.

For Peter the move was a huge success. Two of his best friends lived nearby. Bicycles took them wherever they wanted to go. Peter loved the outdoors and could move through the woods as silently as an Indian. His infinite patience rewarded him with a close acquaintance with all manner of birds and chipmunks who beat a hasty retreat whenever Davey and I approached with Sam crashing about at our heels.

In winter the pond was the scene of spirited hockey games, and in summer Peter and his friends, accompanied by our fish-loving cat, discovered the favorite hiding places of the wily bass. Apparently there was plenty of food for them. Blue-gills were easy to catch, so the cat was seldom disappointed, but bait rarely tempted the bass. We saw one so seldom that I was convinced there were fewer than a dozen in the pond. One winter the ice froze deeper than usual and was covered for several weeks by a heavy blanket of snow. The oxygen beneath it became gradually exhausted, and when the ice melted we were amazed to find fifty-three bass, ranging from ten to fifteen inches in length, floating lifeless on the surface of the water.

In spring there were peeping tree frogs everywhere, but their peeping stopped abruptly whenever we came near them. Even when we sat motionless in their midst, they seemed to know we had not retreated, and never resumed their peeping until we departed. There must have been thousands of the little creatures, but try as I would, I never saw one. As summer wore on hundreds of tadpoles grew into frogs. When we approached the edge of the pond they would splash to safety and watch us pass, only their eyes and the tips of their noses above the water. Later we were lulled to sleep at night by a booming chorus of bullfrogs.

Meanwhile, storm clouds were gathering over the Children's Hospital. Bill Clatworthy's furious outbursts over policies he considered wrong were inexorably isolating him from his sources of support. Though he was sometimes a difficult taskmaster, I had grown to love him and was blind to the strength of his growing opposition. Tom Boles, I felt, supported him loyally, though Bill chose to believe otherwise. The two had never been good friends, and little differences over what I considered minutiae were relentlessly driving them apart. I often wondered if they might have been closer had they been able to find an area of research in which they could work harmoniously together. Instead, they went their separate ways, each caring for his own patients, filling his individual role as a teacher, carrying his defined portion of the administrative load, and pursuing different interests.

Before the storm broke we did share one close moment together. In pooling our efforts to help one little girl I caught a glimpse of what might have been had we succeeded more often in working together toward a single objective.

Like all pediatric surgeons we had been repeatedly frustrated by jaundice in babies. Some of the problems were simple enough. Nearly all babies who became jaundiced on the day of birth had erythroblastosis, caused by Rh incompatibility between their blood and that of their mothers. The use of exchange transfusions had largely solved their problems, and soon it would be possible to prevent erythroblastosis by giving an injection to susceptible mothers. Most babies who became jaundiced a day or two after birth had the self-limited "physiologic" jaundice of the newborn, from which they recovered spontaneously in a few days. An occasional baby suffering from overwhelming infection became jaundiced, but the cause of the illness was usually obvious.

There remained a group of babies who did not have any of these problems, who gradually developed persistent jaundice but appeared otherwise perfectly healthy. They deteriorated so gradually that the change from day to day could barely be noticed. Most lived a year or more before succumbing to advanced liver failure.

One cause of this distressing problem is biliary atresia. In these babies bile cannot leave the liver and make its way to the duodenum because the bile ducts are malformed. Normally, a vast network of ducts runs through the liver, carrying bile to two major branches that emerge from the under surface of the liver and join to form the common bile duct, the trunk of the biliary "tree." From the side of this trunk a single offshoot leads to the gallbladder where part of the bile is stored and concentrated. Bile from the liver drips more or less continually from the end of the common bile duct into the duodenum. When a meal is fed, particularly a meal containing fat, the gallbladder empties, adding to the flow of bile. Bile is rich in bilirubin, a major breakdown product of red blood cells. When the flow of bile is obstructed the patient takes on the deep yellow color known as jaundice.

When a baby with biliary atresia is operated upon, the common bile duct and its two main tributaries can usually be found, but instead of being as big as the baby's little finger, the common duct is a tiny fibrous strand that appears to have no channel within it. Often under the microscope one can see tiny remnants of the passageway, but these are merely vacuoles that do not lead to the liver.

Rarely the abnormality is confined to the portions of the ducts that lie outside the liver. The surgeon may be fortunate enough to find a nubbin of bile duct protruding from the surface of the liver that is sufficiently large to suture to the intestine. In these rare instances, if the operation is performed soon enough after birth, the baby is relieved at once. In his early days at the Boston Children's Hospital beginner's luck favored Dr. Ladd, prompting him to report one of the first cures. He and the surgeons who came after him were dismayed to find how seldom this favorable anatomic circumstance is encountered.

Usually the entire biliary "tree" is abnormal, including its ramifications within the liver. Many surgeons considered these unfortunate babies incurable, justifying an exploratory operation upon them as the only way to find the rare baby who could be helped. A number of Japanese surgeons developed operations that appeared very promising. They identified the remnants of the bile ducts and traced them to the point from which they emerged from the liver. They cut across the ducts at this point and had microscopic examinations made to see if the ducts had any passageway at all within them. Often, even when the duct appeared to be a solid cord, the microscope revealed a tiny channel. If the surgeon thought the channel was large enough he sutured the liver to the intestine so that the little duct could empty into it. If not, he continued upward, dissecting away small bits of liver and patiently examining section after section of tissue under the microscope. The Japanese found that bile would flow from the liver through a duct that was incredibly small. If a duct seventy-five microns in diameter could be found, the baby would slowly become free of jaundice. Seventy-five microns is only ten times the diameter of a single red blood cell.

Here was hope for a group of babies for whom there never had been a ray of hope before, but there were many problems. An adequate flow of bile could be established in only half of the babies. The others were not helped at all. The liver was always severely damaged by the time the operation was performed, since the obstruction had been present long before birth. Many of the babies went on to develop severe cirrhosis with all of its problems, the most dramatic of which is massive hemorrhage from esophageal varices. All in all, the Japanese operations have not often given the glowing long-term results that had been anticipated.

A frequent complication following surgery on the bile ducts is recurring infection of the biliary "tree" known as cholangiolitis. Bile is usually sterile, and the normal junction between the bile duct and the duodenum is designed to resist the entrance of bacteria. These are always present in the intestine, and they find it much easier to invade the bile ducts through a surgically constructed junction than through a natural one. In addition to making the infants ill, recurring attacks of cholangiolitis have a scarring effect on the little ducts, so that after a time they become obstructed by scar tissue and the jaundice returns.

Matters are further complicated by the existence of a medical condition that mimics biliary atresia but is never aided by surgery. It is known as neonatal hepatitis. It differs from the common forms of hepatitis that affect older children and adults. The latter forms are caused by viruses, one moderately contagious, the other transmitted by transfusions of blood from affected people or by reuse of needles that have not been sterilized effectively. If neonatal hepatitis is caused by a virus, it is a virus distinct from the other two in that it never makes adults detectably ill. The mothers of babies with neonatal hepatitis have no jaundice or other evidence of illness and usually have not had the opportunity to acquire a virus through transfusion. The notion that a virus might be at fault is strengthened by the observation that mothers who have given birth to a baby with the disease rarely repeat the calamity, suggesting that they may have sustained a subclinical, or undetectable, infection to which they are subsequently immune. Mothers giving birth to babies with biliary atresia do not often repeat either, and one prominent pathologist has proposed that neonatal hepatitis and biliary atresia may actually be variants of the same ill-defined disease.

From a treatment standpoint the two disorders are very different, as a long and delicate operation offers the only chance to relieve the obstruction of biliary atresia, while prolonged anesthesia and manipulation of the bile ducts cannot possibly help babies with hepatitis. Therefore, it is vitally important to distinguish between the two disorders.

The babies appear virtually identical. Their skin and the whites of their eyes are deep yellow. Since no bile enters the intestine, none appears in the stool. The color of the milk they ingest is almost unchanged, giving rise to stools that are clay colored instead of yellow or brown. The clay referred to is the white clay of which tobacco pipes are made, rather than the dark gray mud that potters use. Blood and serum tests in the two conditions yield identical results. They simply confirm the fact that bile which is ready to leave the liver is prevented from doing so and accumulates in the blood instead.

Many jaundiced babies were subjected to repeated series of blood tests in the hope that a helpful pattern might become discernible, but usually nothing was accomplished except delay. Meanwhile the few babies who could be helped by surgery grew steadily older, approaching the day when even the most skillful operation could no longer help them. The prolonged obstruction to the flow of bile is severely damaging to the liver. An extensive survey of babies with biliary atresia found not a single survivor whose operation had been performed after the age of three months.

Clearly a new way to establish the diagnosis quickly was needed. Bill Clatworthy spelled out a simple solution that was adopted in most pediatric centers around the world. Under his plan jaundiced babies without bile in their stools went directly to the operating room for a very brief operation aimed only at achieving a diagnosis. The operation could be completed in less than ten minutes. An anesthetic of this brief duration could do very little harm to the babies with neonatal hepatitis.

The operation had two objectives. One was to obtain a liver biopsy, a thin wedge of liver tissue that could be studied under the microscope. The second was to introduce a slender tube into the gallbladder so that Hypaque could be injected directly into it. If the baby had hepatitis, the Hypaque would outline small but otherwise normal bile ducts. If the baby had biliary atresia, the Hypaque would remain in the gallbladder, since the bile ducts did not have channels that could carry it away. The x-rays were often conclusive, but sometimes one could not see enough Hypaque to distinguish between the two entities. The microscopic findings in the liver biopsies usually differed markedly, but occasionally did not. By combining the information obtained by both measures one could arrive at the correct diagnosis in most cases.

The beauty of Bill's diagnostic procedure lay in its brevity and simplicity. Pediatricians, aware of the dangers of a long, unnecessary operation on babies who were struggling to recover from hepatitis, were reluctant to turn jaundiced babies over to surgeons until this simple operation was introduced. Thereafter, they gradually came around to accepting the surgeon's help, and the opportunity to help a few babies with biliary atresia improved.

Wennonah was a little black baby whose dark skin obscured the fact that she was jaundiced. When her mother finally convinced her doctor that her eyeballs were dark yellow she was already two months old. She had no trace of bile in her stool, and I took her to the operating room, believing she had either biliary atresia or neonatal hepatitis. I removed a wedge of liver tissue and sutured a small tube into her gallbladder. Both the edge of the liver and the dome of the gallbladder lie just under the abdominal wall. The incision was only about an inch long. The bile ducts cannot be seen through so small an incision. I closed the wound, and she rapidly awoke. We took her to the X-ray Department where Tom Frye watched on the fluoroscope as I injected Hypaque into her gallbladder. Usually only a very small amount can be introduced, and great care must be taken not to force in too much. This time Tom kept calling for more until I had injected more than an ounce of Hypaque. The resulting x-rays showed a round shadow about the size of a golf ball under Wennonah's liver. It was a huge hollow space filled with Hypaque and bile. Wennonah had a choledochal cyst.

Closely related to biliary atresia, perhaps a variant of it, a choledochal cyst is considerably easier to deal with. The ducts within the liver are usually normal, as are the two large ducts that join together at the upper end of the common bile duct. From the side of the common duct a large hollow space develops into which bile flows through a tiny opening. As this balloon-like structure expands it impinges on the side of the common duct, obstructing the flow of bile. When obstruction is present at birth the baby is indistinguishable from those with the more common neonatal hepatitis or biliary atresia.

Though the cyst is often quite large, it may be impossible to feel it when examining the baby. Sometimes, when the infant is given a barium swallow one can see on the x-ray an indentation where the cyst presses on the wall of the duodenum. Sometimes the cyst is discovered when Hypaque is injected into the gallbladder.

The results of surgery for this condition are far from perfect, but much better than for most forms of biliary atresia. The objective is to reduce the size of the cyst by trimming away part of its wall and to suture the remaining edges to the intestine. This I did the day after we obtained our striking x-rays.

Wennonah flourished for a time. Her jaundice cleared completely, she ate eagerly, and grew normally, but she was plagued by repeated bouts of cholangiolitis. The danger of cumulative damage to the bile ducts prompted me to present her case to Bill Clatworthy and Tom Boles at one of our teaching conferences, hoping for a suggestion as to how to prevent further attacks.

Bill led the discussion. As so often happened, there wasn't much left to say when he had summarized his thoughts. He had a genius for getting to the heart of a problem. Cholangiolitis is an infection caused by bacteria. They enter the bile ducts from the small intestine. Usually a steady stream of bile washes them away. If the flow of bile is reduced by an obstruction, invasion of the bile ducts is greatly facilitated. Obstruction, if present in Wennonah, was almost certainly at the point where I had sutured the edges of the cyst wall to the intestine. There is no way to x-ray this critical area.

The decision came down to whether or not Wennonah's attacks of cholangiolitis were severe enough to warrant operating on her, and if so, whether or not we were likely to find an obstruction that could be corrected. Even if we did, what was to prevent future infections? Bill's ingenious mind had come up with a possibility that never in a hundred years would have occurred to the rest of us. Wennonah's appendix would make an ideal conduit to carry bile from the cyst to her intestine!

The fact that an appendix occasionally becomes infected is by no means surprising. What is remarkable is that most never do. Hour after hour, day after day, the lining of the appendix is exposed to millions of bacteria. It must be phenomenally resistant to infection. The appendix has about the same caliber as a normal common bile duct and is long enough to substitute for it. The blood vessels that nourish it are arranged in such a way that the appendix can be moved to its new location. The relatively few bacteria that would gain access to the appendix might easily be controlled by its remarkable powers of resistance. Malcolm Weinberger, our chief resident, had done the operation several times, under Bill's direction, on laboratory animals.

Early one Saturday morning Bill, Tom, and I gathered in the operating room to help Mal operate on Wennonah. If this unusual operation had ever been done before, none of us was aware of it. The operation went along smoothly. I assisted Mal, with Bill and Tom making valuable suggestions as we proceeded.

Through this joint effort Wennonah was greatly improved. Her attacks of cholangiolitis were milder, much less frequent and easier to control.

I felt, and I think the others did too, that the three of us were closer together on that Saturday morning than we had ever been before. If only Bill and Tom could submerge their differences in other joint projects, we could accomplish almost anything.

It was not to be. Bill and the hospital trustees clashed over a series of issues that might have been peacefully resolved. The trustees had the upper hand, and stripped him of his authority as Chief of Pediatric Surgery. When it became clear that the trustees were implacably determined not to reinstate him, Tom became the logical successor. Though he was less imaginative than Bill, and less well known outside Columbus, Tom was eminently qualified, and under his steady, even-handed leadership the department continued to flourish. But all vestiges of friendship and cooperation between Bill and Tom were destroyed, and great possibilities were tragically lost.

39

Cancer

Sidney Farber's demonstration that chemical agents could retard or halt the multiplication of cancer cells had a profound effect on pediatric surgery. Instead of reducing the pediatric surgeon's involvement in caring for children with cancer, chemotherapy greatly increased it. Before drug therapy was introduced, an operation for cancer, sometimes followed by x-ray treatment, either cured the child or was followed by a relentless downhill course. Occasionally, though not very often, after a series of x-ray treatments had caused it to shrink, a tumor could be removed that had been too extensive to resect on the first attempt. Rarely, when a metastasis appeared, could a surgeon cure a child by removing it. A metastasis is a secondary tumor arising from cells cast off from the primary one that have traveled to a new location via the blood or lymph. These cures were rare exceptions, as metastases are usually multiple and defy attempts to remove all of them.

Because of the rapidity with which cancer did its deadly work in children one could be reasonably sure that it was cured if it did not reappear within two years. For some tumors a slightly longer period, defined by Collins' rule, applied. This rule was based on the assumption that any new tumor the child was likely to develop would be of the same type as the original and would grow at the same rate. It took into account the possibility that the original tumor might have begun to grow before the baby was born, perhaps soon after conception. A child who was three years old when his tumor was removed had been conceived three years and nine months earlier. Even if only a single malignant cell were left behind, a tumor arising from it would be expected to become apparent before the child had lived an additional three years and nine months. A few children did develop evidence of recurrence later, but these were rare exceptions. Chemotherapy changed the rules, making it mandatory to follow children much longer.

Tom Boles was ideally suited by ability and temperament to care for children with cancer. He was competent to remove the most extensive tumors that a surgeon could remove, but it was in the after-care and follow-up of children that he really excelled. Nothing upset him more than failure of parents to keep a follow-up appointment. He carefully explained to them why these regular examinations were important and went to great lengths to assure almost perfect compliance. He organized and faithfully supervised a special clinic for children with cancer which all of our patients regularly attended. Together with Bill Newton and other oncologists, the experts in chemotherapy, Tom saw to it that all details of the treatment protocols were carried out on time.

Different forms of cancer require different treatment, as do different stages of the same disease. The protocols are designed to assure that treatment schedules appropriate for each child are followed. They are formulated by groups of pediatric surgeons, radiotherapists, and oncologists representing the major pediatric centers in the United States and Canada and are designed so that children in several institutions can be treated in an identical manner. No child is denied a form of treatment that has been proven beneficial. If the entire tumor can and should be removed, this is always done. If x-ray therapy is known to be helpful, it is always given. X-ray treatment can be harmful, and no one wants to give it if it is not necessary. The only way to find out if the harmful effects outweigh the benefits in a given situation is to divide truly comparable patients into two groups, giving x-ray therapy to one and not the other. By pooling large numbers of patients the answer can be rapidly obtained and the fewest children harmed before the issue is settled. The same is

282   A GIFT OF COURAGE

true of the anticancer drugs. They all have potentially harmful
effects and should be given for the shortest time in the smallest
and most efficiently spaced doses that will accomplish their desired effects. Great scientific care must go into designing the
protocols, and great moral care as well, to ensure that they give
promise of doing the greatest good and the least harm. Once
agreed upon they must be rigidly adhered to by all participating surgeons, x-ray therapists, and oncologists.

There are accepted avenues of escape. Should a particular
child develop a condition warranting a different form of treatment, he can be withdrawn from a protocol at any time. Judgment in doing this is essential because if all children were withdrawn, the objective could never be achieved, but no child must
be harmed by adhering to a protocol that no longer fits his
needs. As soon as a protocol yields statistically valid results its
less-effective alternative is abandoned. The number of children
treated according to each protocol varies and cannot be prede-
termined. If one alternative is minimally superior to the other,
many children must be treated before the difference becomes apparent. If one regimen is far more effective, only a few children
must be treated before this becomes obvious.

The information gathered by physicians treating adults is carefully scrutinized, but often this information is not relevant to
children because they suffer from very different forms of cancer.
The common cancers in adults, arising in the breast, lung, stomach, and colon, are almost never seen in children. Wilms' tumor,
by far the most common malignancy affecting children's kidneys, is very rare in adults. The kidney cancer of adults is an entirely different disease. The same is true of neuroblastoma, the
common adrenal tumor of childhood. Physicians caring for children must develop their own information, as neuroblastoma is
practically never seen in adults. The cooperation between representatives of the major children's medical centers is truly remarkable and represents a bright chapter in the history of child care.
Many children are alive and well because of it.

In large institutions it is neither feasible nor wise to limit the
surgical care of all cancer patients to one surgeon. At the same
time, one surgeon must play a dominant role in assuring that all
the surgeons understand the protocols and adhere to them. Tom

Boles and Bill Newton conducted weekly tumor conferences which we all attended. Every new cancer patient was carefully discussed. His history and physical findings were presented, and if he had been operated upon, the surgeon described what he had found at the operation and what he had done about it. Microscopic slides of the tumor were projected on a screen and described in detail by a pathologist so that everyone could see and hear the reasons for determining the type of tumor under discussion. This diagnosis is critically important, for it determines whether or not x-ray therapy should be used and how much radiation will be needed. The choice of drug or combination of drugs also depends on the type of tumor.

Equally important is the extent to which the cancer has spread. X-rays, body scans, and bone marrow examinations contribute to this evaluation, as do the findings at the time of operation. The protocols describe this spread in a series of stages. The stages vary in detail from one type of tumor to another, but in general, stage I describes tumors that have been completely removed, while stage IV describes cancer that has spread throughout the body, beyond the reach of both surgeon and radiotherapist. The criteria for these stages are constantly being updated as new knowledge is acquired.

The tumor conferences at which we discussed our many children with cancer sometimes gave rise to heated debates, but we were nearly always able to reach an acceptable consensus. As a result of these conferences we were able to offer our patients a standard of care that none of us, working independently, could hope to achieve.

Susan came to my office late one afternoon with a lump in her neck. She was a slender, athletic teenager who played trumpet in her high school marching band. She gave every appearance of being in perfect health. The lump was very firm and smooth, causing only a slight bulge in the skin overlying it. Though I could feel only a small portion of its surface, I had the impression that it resembled a hen's egg whose major portion lay deep in her neck, protected from my examining fingers by her collar bone. It was not at all tender and had never caused the slightest twinge of pain. Susan had been aware of its presence for at least a few days, but was not sure when she had first noticed it. With the exception of this solitary bump I could find absolutely nothing wrong with her.

I sent her to the hospital for x-rays of her neck and chest. Her father was with her, having left work early to bring her to my office. When I suggested that the x-rays be obtained at once his facial expression did not change, but from the look in his eyes I saw that I had frightened him nearly out of his wits. In spite of his outwardly calm appearance he was one of the most apprehensive fathers with whom I ever dealt. The events of the next few days would have ruffled the equanimity of the most stoic parent. He was a wreck before they were over.

I had secretly hoped that the x-rays might reveal the presence of a cervical rib. An occasional child is born with a rudimentary extra rib above the usual twelve, sometimes on one side, sometimes on both. They seldom cause any problems and usually should be left alone. I had once been rescued from operating unnecessarily on a little girl with a cervical rib by an alert intern who spotted it on an x-ray moments before the anesthetist began to put her to sleep. The fact that the little girl's father was a physician would have added an extra dimension to my embarrassment. Thereafter I always looked for cervical ribs, but I never saw another child with one.

Susan did not have a cervical rib. The mass in her neck cast only a faint shadow. Though it felt hard, it was not bone. Her chest x-ray showed that the lump in her neck was not her only problem. In the upper part of her chest was a wide shadow undoubtedly caused by some sort of abnormal mass. On the lateral view of her chest one could see that the mass was about equidistant from her spine and her breastbone. Masses in this location are usually clusters of enlarged lymph nodes. The mass I could feel in Susan's neck was contiguous with that in her chest and was probably also a lymph node. One might hope that some form of chronic infection like tuberculosis was responsible, but this was highly unlikely without some x-ray evidence of infection in the lungs. Susan's lungs appeared perfectly normal. Reluctantly I admitted what I had known all along. Susan almost certainly had Hodgkin's disease.

Hodgkin's disease is a form of cancer that originates in the lymphatic system. Lymph is a slightly turbid fluid that arises in the spaces between body cells and makes its way slowly toward the heart through a network of nearly invisible channels known as lymphatic ducts. Along the way the lymph passes through one or more lymph nodes, little nubbins of specialized tissue that serve as filtering stations. Here bacteria or other harmful substances are removed from the lymph and destroyed.

Normal lymph nodes are quite small, the largest resembling small beans. Most are not palpable, even if they lie directly beneath the skin. Rapid enlargement, particularly if the enlarging nodes are painful or tender, is usually a response to infection. Enlarged, tender nodes in the neck frequently accompany tonsillitis. The enlargement regresses when the infection subsides, though often the nodes remain somewhat larger than they were originally, and sometimes can be felt in the neck for years.

Lymph nodes also filter out wandering cancer cells. Probably most are destroyed, but if a malignant cell survives and begins to multiply, the lymph node becomes the site of a metastasis. The presence of a malignant tumor deep within the body can sometimes be detected by biopsying an enlarged lymph node lying beneath the skin. Often, though not always, the tumor cells in the lymph node retain the characteristics of the primary cancer, making it possible to determine the organ in which it lurks.

In Hodgkin's disease the malignancy does not arise in cells brought to the node from a tumor elsewhere in the body. Rather, it appears to represent a change in cells normally present in lymph nodes. The disease is believed to begin in a single node or group of contiguous nodes. If unchecked it gradually spreads, first to other groups of nodes and eventually to tissues beyond the lymphatic system. Favorite early targets are the spleen, liver, and bone marrow.

At first, patients with Hodgkin's disease feel perfectly well. As the disease progresses they may experience chills and periodic fevers accompanied by feelings of weakness and fatigue. They may lose weight and develop anemia. Their ability to combat infection is progressively impaired. Some complain of severe itching or of pains in their legs, back, or abdomen. Susan had none of these complaints.

The first step was to prove conclusively that Hodgkin's disease was what she really had. This I did the morning after I first met her by removing a sliver of tissue from the mass in her neck. Under the microscope we could see the distorted architecture of a lymph node crowded with the abnormal cells of Hodgkin's disease.

The next step was to define the limits to which the disease had spread. The malignant cells are very sensitive to radiation. It is important to irradiate all affected nodes during the initial course of treatment. This has been shown to be far superior to chasing the disease hither and yon, treating one limited area after another as evidence of its relentless spread appears.

The lymph nodes in the armpits are intimately connected to those in the neck and chest. Spread to these nodes is so often seen that they are routinely included in the field of radiation when the disease arises in the neck. The real question was how far below the chest it had spread. The shoulders and armpits can be radiated with little risk, but we did not wish to subject the abdominal organs to x-ray therapy without knowing that the lymph nodes within the abdomen were involved. There are many groups of nodes in the abdomen, pelvis, and groin. In a patient as slender as Susan enlarged nodes in the groin would have been readily palpable. Had they been filled with malignant cells we could be reasonably sure that the nodes in her abdomen were also involved, but we could feel no swelling in her groin.

We performed a lymphangiogram, a procedure in which a radiopaque substance is injected into a lymphatic vessel at the base of the toes. From here it travels slowly toward the heart. On the way some of it is filtered out by the nodes in the groin, pelvis, and abdomen. On x-rays taken a few hours later one can see the opaque material lodged in the nodes. Normal nodes appear small and uniformly opacified. Abnormal nodes appear much larger and may show a patchy distribution of the opaque material. Lymphangiograms are helpful but are sometimes plagued by technical difficulties and at best give only circumstantial evidence. We saw nothing definitely abnormal in Susan's lymphangiogram.

The only sure way to establish the presence or absence of Hodgkin's disease within the abdomen is to perform what is known as a staging laparotomy. This is a major operation involving removal of all or a part of the spleen, biopsying the liver, and removing representative nodes from four to six specific locations. If a bone marrow biopsy has not been done beforehand, it may be included in the staging laparotomy. All of the removed tissue is carefully studied under the microscope.

Despite her robust appearance, the operation affected Susan as if she had been struck in the abdomen by a giant hammer. For two or three days she seemed almost totally immobilized, as if convinced she would suffer great pain if she made the slightest attempt to move. She insisted that she felt pretty well, but like her apprehensive father she was consumed by fears she was unable to vocalize. When I convinced her that the microscope had shown no evidence of disease within her abdomen she finally relaxed and after sleeping soundly for several hours convalesced rapidly, at least in a physical sense. Her confidence had been dealt a staggering blow. Having felt perfectly normal when she came to the hospital for what she thought would be only an x-ray of her neck, it was a long time before she could return without being fearful that the hospital would suddenly engulf her again.

Guided by the information we compiled from her x-rays and her operation, the x-ray therapist was able to irradiate all involved lymph nodes as well as those in a limited area beyond them. When the radiation was finished Susan underwent a course of chemotherapy using a combination of four powerful drugs. From her high school marching band she went on to play the French horn in the Columbus Symphony Orchestra, and is now pursuing her musical career in graduate school. It will require a lifetime to prove that she is permanently free of this mysterious disease that was nearly always fatal until she was old enough to start kindergarten. Patients like Susan, treated in the earliest stages of Hodgkin's disease, now appear to have a 90 percent chance of living normal lives.

40

When the Lights Burn Brightly

A favorite theme of commencement speakers is that much of the information the graduates have toiled so hard to learn has already become obsolete. Medical students must assimilate a staggering array of facts, but they are exhorted to regard their learning experiences primarily as a series of exercises in medical problem solving. The ultimate goal of medical education is held to be the ability to make appropriate decisions based upon new facts as they emerge. Before taking the oath of Hippocrates new physicians are reminded for at least the hundredth time to be wary of statistics, as statistical data can easily be used to "prove" statements that are not true. At the same time they are urged to continue to read throughout their professional lives, being ruthlessly selective, as the mass of printed medical knowledge is said to double about every two years.

Despite the difficulties in keeping abreast of reliable new medical knowledge, most doctors find it infinitely easier to do this than to perceive and react appropriately to creeping changes in social, moral, and ethical values. Many more surgeons know how to turn on and adjust the newest mechanical respirator than are sure of when it is "right" to turn it off.

Just what does "Thou shalt not kill" really mean? Far from

learning the answer in medical school, most medical students, at least in my day, never heard the issue discussed. Is it always wrong for one human being to take the life of another? Apparently not. Most people who abhor killing condone it when it is done in self-defense. Whose life is more valuable than whose? If killing an unborn baby is the only way to save the life of the mother, is it always right to do so? Is it ever morally permissible to give a lethal dose of morphine to a patient in agony from an incurable disease? Many humane physicians did so in years past, secure in the belief that it was appropriate. Many of today's physicians think so too, though far fewer would dare to act on their conviction. It has become increasingly easier to discern what constitutes malpractice than what is right.

Slowly but surely society has moved away from the belief that the wise physician is best qualified to make some of these difficult decisions. As our technical abilities increased we physicians have been perceived more and more as cold, ruthless scientists whom other elements of society must keep in check. Are the judges in our courts truly better qualified than physicians? Do they, as individuals, have fewer opinions or prejudices? What of the clergy? The Catholic Church maintains that in hopeless situations it is not necessary to apply extraordinary measures. Many feel this is eminently reasonable. In principle it may be, but who is to declare a situation hopeless, and who is to determine what constitutes extraordinary or heroic measures?

As practicing pediatric surgeons, we are protected by the age limits of our patients from the necessity of making some of the ethical decisions that plague our colleagues. We may have opinions as to the propriety of abortion, but are never faced with having to decide whether or not to perform one. We are never called upon to make decisions regarding prolonging the life of the elderly. Like other physicians, we have often been able to hide in indecision or delay until death quickly settled an issue without our intervention.

One tragically frequent occurrence presents us with an inescapable dilemma. A number of babies with Down's syndrome are born with duodenal atresia. Down's syndrome, also known as mongolism, invariably imposes severe intellectual limitations on its little victims. A few at the lower end of the scale can truly be described as imbeciles. Most are capable of learning, and can accomplish far more if given competent, specialized education than if left to compete with normal children, but self-sufficiency in an unsheltered world is beyond expectation for even the brightest child with Down's syndrome.

Some of these unfortunate infants are born with duodenal atresia, a congenital malformation causing complete obstruction of the intestine that is always fatal if not relieved by a surgical operation. Both in mongols and in normal infants the operation is very simple and almost always results in permanent relief. From a surgical point of view, duodenal atresia offers a classically clear choice between certain death and uncomplicated survival.

Does mongolism constitute a hopeless situation in which extraordinary measures can properly be withheld? If so, is a relatively simple operation with a predictably successful outcome an extraordinary measure? Certainly, if the baby did not have Down's syndrome, the operation would always be performed. Who has the right to decide? The parents? The surgeon? A hospital ethics committee? Society? Is there an absolute answer, or do individual considerations apply? Does the fact that one mother facing this decision has four normal children while another has none have any bearing on the issue? What if a mother with no other children is nearing the end of her reproductive years, with little hope of conceiving again? What if the parents lack resources to provide the extra education so important to achieving the baby's limited intellectual potential? Is it "right" to save the life of a baby who is doomed to life-long dependence on society?

When I began my practice it was customary for the surgeon to discuss these considerations with the parents and leave the decision to them. In doing so I always hoped that I painted an accurate, unbiased picture of the baby's outlook. Parents often welcomed my suggestion that they consult their pastor or priest. Despite the convictions these troubled clergymen must have held, I was repeatedly impressed by their restraint. Nearly always they reassured the parents that the decision was theirs to make, and that in the days and months ahead their church would support them regardless of what they chose to do. Sometimes grandparents and other family members were consulted. This could be inconvenient, as it often prolonged the agony of indecision, but I think it rarely changed the outcome.

If the decision was made to go ahead with the operation, the parents were usually greatly relieved and things went very smoothly. As quickly as possible I put them in touch with other parents who had made the same decision, and these couples were always helpful and supportive. The baby usually remained in the hospital for two to three weeks and then went home. For the first few months he behaved so like other babies that the parents usually believed his intellect was going to be normal. Gradually the mothers, and later the fathers, reluctantly began to recognize the truth as their baby's performance lagged farther and farther behind.

If the parents decided against the operation, they were subject to a long period of mounting anxiety. Death did not come quickly. The baby languished for at least two weeks before succumbing. During this time it was essential for doctors and nurses to act in a uniformly supportive way, as many of the parents visited their dying babies every day. A number of couples reversed their decisions and implored me to perform the operation they had formerly declined. I never refused, though often the chance to save the baby's life had slipped to a fraction of its original potential. One little baby who had starved for many days died shortly after his fatally delayed operation. The suffering of his parents was perhaps the most intense I ever witnessed. I was certain I would never see them again, but a year later they came to see me, bringing a beautiful, healthy baby girl.

Public opinion changed as the years passed, so gradually that those of us who were caught up in the daily work of child care were scarcely aware of its implications. Child abuse and neglect were becoming more widely recognized. More and more frequently we found ourselves in the role of advocate for the child, pleading with the courts to free little victims from the tyranny of their abusing parents. Students of child abuse assured us that much of the apparent increase was not due to a rise in the number of battered children but to heightened social awareness that brought more of them to light. Whatever the cause, abused and neglected children appeared in greatly increasing numbers, and the right, indeed the duty, of society to protect them became widely accepted.

This loss of faith in the right of parents to sole authority over their children had an unexpected result. The right of parents to decide against an operation for duodenal atresia began to be challenged. To deny the procedure now is widely held to be a form of parental neglect. Regardless of the wishes of the parents or the convictions of the surgeon, society has made it essentially impossible to withhold the operation.

I really do not know whether this change in social perception approaches or retreats from what is truly right. History does not show that surrender of parents' rights to the state has always been beneficial to children. We may be witnessing just the beginning of more sweeping changes in the same direction, or the pendulum may be about to swing back toward the values of an earlier day. Only time will tell.

The distressing intellectual limitation of Down's syndrome may soon yield to research on the chemistry of the brain. When it does, one moral dilemma, easy to define but difficult to resolve, will simply disappear. On that day, perhaps not too far off, literally thousands of intellectually deprived people will awaken to new levels of awareness, some in their infancy, some during childhood, some toward the end of their lives. Will they be happier when the lights in their minds burn brightly than when they flickered under mongolism's smothering blanket? Now, for the first time, they too will be called upon to deal with moral dilemmas. God help them, for they will be more bewildered than Rip Van Winkle, who awoke one morning to find he had slumbered for twenty years while the world went on without him.

41

Malpractice

Every time I go to the airport I see something I wish we had in hospitals. It is a little booth where a passenger can buy insurance that pays his family a specified amount if he fails to arrive at his destination alive. This compensation is based entirely on the result, without regard for the cause of the accident. The airplane manufacturer may or may not be at fault. The maintenance crew may or may not have done its job properly. The pilot may or may not have made an avoidable error. It doesn't matter. The passenger was harmed; his family receives compensation. Liability insurance, which the airline purchases, pays only if guilt or negligence can be proved, usually through a lawsuit. Both types of insurance are appropriate for passengers embarking on air travel. It seems to me that both types should be provided for patients about to undergo major surgery.

As matters stand now, patients cannot receive compensation for a bad result unless the surgeon can be proven guilty of malpractice. There is no question that some surgeons do deserve to be sued for blunders or neglect, but patients are sometimes harmed when neither stupidity nor negligence is responsible. Occasionally the lawyers who represent them are avaricious rogues who deserve to be sued themselves, but not always. More than a few honest lawyers believe their clients deserve compensation and seek to obtain it for them the only way they can, by suing the doctor. Sometimes they are spectacularly successful. Judgments in excess of a million dollars still make headlines, but they are not as rare as they used to be.

As the number of successful suits increased, many insurance companies were forced to withdraw from the malpractice field, sometimes refusing to renew coverage of surgeons they had served for twenty or thirty years. In the late nineteen seventies it became extremely difficult for new surgeons, even those graduating from the leading surgical training programs, to obtain any coverage at all. Doctors complained about the rising cost of malpractice insurance as if they paid for it. They don't. They merely pass the cost on to the patient in the form of higher fees.

The cost of malpractice insurance is only the tip of the iceberg. Doctors were forced, or perceived that they were forced, to practice "defensive medicine," ordering thousands of unnecessary or marginally necessary x-rays and laboratory tests, not for the patient's benefit but to make his medical chart look good. The staggering costs of these extra tests are usually thought to be paid by health insurance companies, but of course they are not. Like malpractice premiums, these costs are passed on to the patient.

It would be far simpler to deal with the problem of "unnecessary" tests if medical progress stood still while the legal and insurance industries caught up, but medical progress does not stand still. Diagnostic procedures that only a short time ago were confined to research centers have now become so commonplace that it is no longer farsighted to use them but downright essential. The classic example is the CAT scan.

CAT stands for computerized axial tomography, a sophisticated and very expensive form of x-ray evaluation. When this spectacular advance became available nearly all large hospitals rushed to buy the costly scanning equipment and hire the required additional trained personnel. Many people considered the CAT scanner an expensive luxury. It was widely held that only one hospital in a large city should have one and that the very few patients for whom its use was indicated should all go there. Like most new inventions, the CAT scanner is unquestionably overused at times, but its value has exceeded the wildest dreams of most of us who read the early reports about it. It has revolutionized neurosurgery to such an extent that no neurosurgeon can function without it. Often the critical status of the patient who needs the scanner makes him unlikely to survive transportation from one hospital to another. Except in very small hospitals the technique has become a medical and surgical necessity. In many critical situations, failure to use it is malpractice.

For several reasons pediatric surgeons are not sued very often. Perhaps the most important reason is that their patients are not breadwinners. The need for compensation when they are disabled is not as great as it can be for adults. In addition, children are inherently healthy, with incredible powers of recovery. Given half a chance, they tend to get well. Parents are prone to seek attention more quickly for their children than for themselves, so that children's disorders are apt to be treated at an early stage when recovery is most likely.

A large percentage of pediatric surgeons work in teaching hospitals where their work is constantly scrutinized. Many a surgeon has been saved from embarrassment by a questioning medical student or intern, as I was by the intern who spotted the cervical rib I had overlooked on the x-ray. Mistakes tend not to be repeated in an atmosphere in which every patient is discussed on teaching rounds or in conferences with pathologists, radiologists, or other specialists. The new information reported in medical and surgical journals cannot be ignored in a teaching hospital. The exacting system of medical record-keeping offers the lawyer few opportunities to argue negligence because of the detail with which all aspects of care are documented. A complete, accurate medical record is the best defense a surgeon can present in a court of law.

Perhaps equally important is the attitude of the parents. They tend to believe that bringing their child to a major medical center offers him the best chance for recovery. When the child does not survive they are likely to believe that if the medical center could not save him, probably he couldn't have been saved anywhere else either.

I had only one brush with the threat of a malpractice suit, an experience that illustrates the shortcomings of our system of compensation based upon the necessity of establishing guilt. I was just finishing the paperwork in my office one afternoon when Helen announced that Cy Wolske was on the phone. Cy

Wolske was the lawyer most feared by doctors in Columbus because he had a well-deserved reputation for winning malpractice suits against them.

A few weeks earlier I had removed an apparently innocuous lump from the neck of a little three-year-old girl. It was about the size of a cherry, darker and redder than the fat that surrounded it. It did not look in any way unusual. We removed several small midline masses from children's necks every year. Almost always they were thyroglossal duct cysts. These are congenital malformations associated with the development of the thyroid gland. Although present at birth, they often are not noticed until they have enlarged considerably, usually in the second or third year of life. They rarely cause serious trouble, but are somewhat disfiguring and difficult to hide because they lie just below the Adam's apple in the center of the neck. Occasionally one of them becomes infected, causing both family and physician to wish it had been removed earlier.

This lump was not a thyroglossal duct cyst. The microscopic report, which I received two days after the operation, revealed thyroid tissue instead, and subsequent tests indicated that after I removed the malformation the little girl had no remaining thyroid tissue at all. She would have to take thyroid pills for the rest of her life.

Unquestionably she had been harmed. Her parents, and later she and her husband, would face a lifetime of inconvenience and medical expense as a result of this misadventure. One could make a strong argument that they deserved financial compensation.

The little girl and her mother came to my office where I explained what had happened and what they would have to do about it. It was not a complete disaster, as thyroid replacement is easy to manage and relatively inexpensive. Nevertheless, I was deeply saddened to have inflicted this injury on her. The mother appreciated my discomfort and reassured me that she considered it an honest mistake for which she did not blame me at all. She would explain the problem to her husband, and they would take their daughter to an endocrinologist as I advised.

The father was understandably upset, though he did not communicate his feelings to me. He consulted a lawyer, who told him he did not think he could win a malpractice suit against me.

Instead of accepting this advice, the father cast about in search of a lawyer who would win.

I had never met Cy Wolske, though I had heard other surgeons grumble about his tenacity. I was prepared for a very unpleasant and possibly damaging experience, but it did not turn out that way. When he explained that he was gathering information on which to decide whether or not to prosecute me I invited him to come to my office to discuss the case. My colleagues were horrified. That is not the way it is supposed to work. "Never talk to a lawyer whom you have not retained. The scoundrel will trick you into making all sorts of statements that he will later use against you." If I heard it once I heard it a dozen times. It was nonsense.

Cy came to the office, read all my records, and discussed the case at length with me. I had done the conventional examinations and documented the results. I had not done a radioactive isotope scan. This simple, inexpensive, and completely painless examination would have forestalled the tragedy by showing the absence of thyroid tissue in its usual location on either side of the midline. All of the radioactive substance usually avidly assimilated by thyroid tissue would have been concentrated in the lump I proposed to remove.

The scan was relatively new at the time this little girl was treated, but it could not have been considered still experimental. I could easily have had one made. The issue was not whether or not I could have obtained the study but whether or not my failure to do so constituted malpractice.

The standard by which malpractice suits are decided is whether or not the doctor's actions conform to the usual care exercised by other physicians in the community. Originally the "community" was construed as relatively small, allowing different standards to apply in rural areas from those in large cities. More recently the "community" has been expanded to include the whole United States, the reasoning being that experts as far away as Boston, Miami, San Diego, and Seattle are all within easy reach by telephone. Thus, the question was not whether Bill and Tom would have been expected to obtain a scan, but whether a majority of the nation's pediatric surgeons would have done so.

At that time only a small minority of pediatric surgeons would have used a radioactive isotope scan to study every child with a midline neck mass. Cy informed his client that he could not win a malpractice suit against me, and the father abandoned his quest for compensation. Since then the use of the scan has become nearly universal, perhaps hastened by the threat of legal harassment, perhaps purely because its value has been widely recognized. Should similar circumstances arise today, a malpractice suit would almost certainly be successful.

There is scant cause for joy in this little girl's story. It is true that my reputation was not tarnished by the unpleasant publicity that attends malpractice suits. My license to practice was not revoked. My malpractice insurance premium was not raised, nor was my coverage terminated as it sometimes is when litigation goes against the doctor. But a little girl was hurt by an operation that was supposed to help her, and her family was denied compensation that a fairer system might have provided.

The booth at the airport may not symbolize a system that would fit the needs of patients who are harmed by the efforts of their doctors. Perhaps there is a better way for patients to pay directly for insurance against an untoward result. Workmen's compensation systems, in which the award is automatic and depends upon the degree of disability without regard to guilt or innocence, may come closer to what is required. There is a need, and until it is filled millions of dollars will continue to be squandered in lawyers' fees and in excessive x-rays and laboratory tests. Doctors will continue to practice "defensive medicine," treating hospital charts instead of patients.

When the need is filled, neither malpractice nor the need to insure against it will disappear. True instances of malpractice will continue to occur and should be vigorously prosecuted. But the judgments will be much more reasonable when proving the doctor guilty is no longer the *only* way to compensate his patients.

42

Something Had to Be Done

In 1978 fifty thousand infants and children were treated in our Emergency Department. The number of patients was increasing, not only in ours, but in Emergency Departments everywhere. Fewer and fewer practitioners were keeping office hours in the evening or on weekends. House calls were becoming ancient history. The alternatives to the Emergency Department were disappearing, and the trend was irreversible because the reasons for it were valid and compelling. The hospital Emergency Department offered many advantages, including abundant nursing help, readily available laboratory and x-ray facilities, and an array of specialized equipment that physicians could not provide in their offices or in their patients' homes.

It became fashionable to grumble about the minor complaints with which people came to the Emergency Department. Many were not true emergencies. Often a doctor could determine with a few simple questions and a brief examination that a child could safely have waited until morning. Unfortunately, doctors do not decide when it is necessary to take children to the Emergency Department. Parents do.

One of the loudest complainers was Miner Seymour. Miner was an experienced, conscientious pediatrician and a pretty good sport as well. Observing that he did not actually spend much time in the Emergency Department, I dared him one evening to screen a hundred consecutive episodes that had prompted parents to bring their children there. By his own count, fewer than 10 percent of these parents could have been expected to know that their children did not require prompt attention. Like it or not, hospitals had no choice but to gear up to meet the relentlessly increasing demand for emergency medical services.

Different hospitals responded in different ways. Some required of every doctor on the staff a specified number of hours of service in the Emergency Department. This worked reasonably well until the staff dermatologist missed a diagnosis of meningitis or other serious medical problem for which his training had not prepared him. Other hospitals assigned responsibility for all emergency patients to groups of physicians who specialized in emergency medicine. In many non-teaching hospitals this resulted in better care, but the system was difficult to reconcile with the needs of teaching hospitals where emergency work is essential to the training of interns and residents.

Young physicians endure the long hours and grueling work of internship and residency in order to gain an education. In doing so they give a great deal of service, but giving service is not their primary goal. In our hospital they were providing nearly all of the emergency care for a thousand children a week. Treating innumerable runny noses and suturing hundreds of little cuts eventually cease to be meaningful learning experiences. Something had to be done to lighten their load while preserving for them the opportunity to treat as many serious emergency conditions as possible under supervision before they entered practice and had to go it alone.

In most Emergency Departments half of the patients arrive between the hours of three in the afternoon and eleven at night. Ours was no exception. During these busy hours we set up a separate Emergency Department for minor problems. This was staffed by practicing pediatricians who were assisted by a separate group of nurses and medical students. Patients were triaged, or sorted, by a nurse. Patient flow was greatly speeded by this simple arrangement, and the morale of the pediatric residents was tremendously improved. With some of the pressure relieved, they became more effective teachers, so that the medical students who worked with them also benefited.

For the surgeons a somewhat different approach was required.

They were inundated with minor lacerations. On a busy weekend it was not unusual for sixty children to come to the Emergency Department for repair of one or more cuts requiring only a few sutures and a small dressing. Despite their simplicity, these little cuts required an inordinate amount of time to treat properly. Children cannot be rushed into painful or frightening treatment.

The hospital employed as orderlies a number of men who had served as hospital corpsmen in the armed forces. These technicians had received training and acquired skills that they were not allowed to use in civilian life. I saw in them an answer to a very pressing problem, provided I could find a legal way to employ them. Nowhere in Ohio could I find a single hospital that permitted anyone other than a licensed physician to suture lacerations. Clearly, to do so would not be conventional practice, the mainstay of defense against malpractice suits.

I first had to satisfy all doubters that the technicians received appropriate formal training to prepare them for their new role. With the help of Ron Berggren, the university's Chief of Plastic Surgery, I designed a curriculum that reviewed their military training and emphasized the special needs of children. These included proper sedation and safe, comfortable physical restraint as well as protection against infections of all sorts, including tetanus. Ron drilled them in suturing technique, supervising a number of sessions during which they practiced repairing jagged lacerations in the skin of pigs' feet obtained from a meat packing plant. John Garvin, our Chief of Anesthesia, taught them the safe use of Xylocaine, a rapidly acting local anesthetic similar to Novocain. When the course was completed the technicians sutured a number of children's lacerations with Ron or me acting as assistant, teacher, and supervisor.

The hospital attorney drew up a document which the parents were required to sign in addition to the regular consent-to-treatment form. My heart sank when I first saw it. It was as complicated as the front page of a will, and I was sure no parent would sign it. It carefully identified the technician, clearly stating that he was not a physician but a trained technician working under the supervision of a physician. It identified the child and the number and location of his wounds. Finally, it bore the signature of the parent, signifying that he or she understood what was proposed and agreed to it. Like all medical-consent forms, it was open to challenge in court, but it represented an honest attempt to obtain and record an "informed" consent. Despite its complexity, fewer than one parent in twenty declined to sign it.

Most of the children would be going to their own physicians for removal of their sutures. It was imperative that these doctors understand what we proposed to do. To my surprise, none of the more than four hundred physicians I contacted raised any objection to including their patients in this new program. After it was underway the only complaint they voiced was the welcome one that the sutures were finer than those placed by doctors in other hospitals—and therefore more difficult to remove.

In the surgical clinic I had an opportunity to see a number of healed lacerations and thus was able to exercise a measure of "quality control." The technicians' results more than justified my faith in them. They had a natural rapport with frightened children and could talk even the most hysterical youngster into peaceful submission. They depended far less on sedation and physical restraint than did the average intern or resident. Children and parents loved these gentle, patient technicians. Many young doctors learned from them secrets of dealing with children's fears which cannot be discovered in textbooks or lectures.

Meanwhile the number of hospitals employing full-time emergency physicians was rapidly increasing. The early positions were filled by "second career" physicians who had tired of the irregular hours and other demands of private practice. Gradually young physicians in training began to see emergency medicine as a challenge and began to demand formal training in the specialty. To meet this demand a number of special training programs sprang up across the country. Most of them accepted applicants who had completed at least a year of internship and often a year or two of residency. Thereafter the trainees spent two or three years in a concentrated exposure to all forms of medical and surgical emergencies. All of the programs concentrated primarily on adults. Pediatrics and pediatric surgery were usually not given sufficient emphasis. Ideally, program directors should appoint trained pediatric emergency specialists to their faculties, but where were these people to come from?

Our large Emergency Department could easily accommodate four candidates who wanted to become teachers of pediatric emergency medicine. We began with four senior residents who had completed the training requirements for board certification as pediatricians. It was immediately apparent that their previous training had equipped them better to handle medical than surgical emergencies. They already knew a great deal of pediatric medicine. Their exposure to the various pediatric surgical specialties had been quite limited.

The job of coordinating the teaching efforts of the surgical specialists fell to me. Included were representatives from anesthesia, dentistry, ophthalmology, orthopedics, ear, nose and throat, neurosurgery, thoracic surgery, plastic surgery, and urology, as well as our own Department of General Pediatric Surgery. Fortunately, they all believed in the importance of the project and were more than willing to help. Each specialist analyzed what he could offer and how it could best be presented.

The anesthetists took our trainees into the operating room for two weeks of drill in the fundamentals of respiration, including insertion of breathing tubes and management of respirators. After this tour in the operating room respiratory emergencies held little terror for them.

An amazing number of babies and children, nearly eight thousand a year, came to the Emergency Department with ear, nose, and throat problems. Herb Birck, who headed the ENT Department, was so dynamic and enthusiastic that he was repeatedly voted the most effective teacher in the program. Another surprise, at least to me, was the number of children with dental emergencies. Nearly six thousand children a year came to the Emergency Department with toothaches, infections, or dental injuries. Many of these could be handled, at least initially, by physicians, but some required immediate skilled dental care if one or more teeth were to be saved. Ned Kramer was delighted to have an opportunity to teach pediatricians the fundamentals of emergency dental care, a subject completely foreign to them.

Among the most frightening of all emergencies are those involving loss of consciousness. Often decisive action by emergency physicians in the first few moments after injury can be more important to brain-injured patients than anything a neurosurgeon can do for them later. Pete Sayers took the trainees onto the neurosurgical service for an extended period during which they had an opportunity to follow the progress of children recovering from head injuries.

Fractures, sprains, and muscle injuries are very common in children. Often the x-rays clearly show broken bones, but in small children certain fractures are easily missed. Sometimes success is obtained only by suspecting a specific kind of injury and ordering the exact x-ray views that can bring it to light. Ed Eyring conducted a busy fracture clinic which the trainees attended every week. Here he discussed the mechanisms of injury that caused children's bones to break in certain ways so that the proper questions could be asked and the proper examinations made. Tom Frye spent an hour with the Emergency Department staff every day and went over with them all of the x-rays taken during the previous twenty-four hours. This intensive course in radiology paid handsome dividends. Very few x-ray diagnoses were missed by the emergency physicians in the middle of the night while the staff radiologists were at home in bed. Missing a diagnosis on an x-ray is always embarrassing, and sometimes in emergency situations can have very serious consequences.

For my own part, I emphasized the surgical emergencies of the newborn, the various surgical causes of abdominal pain, and the treatment of burns and other injuries. When they completed their training the four young doctors knew more about more kinds of childhood emergencies than many pediatricians learn in a lifetime.

To help my teaching I drew up and published a set of guidelines for the initial care of the injured child. This was relatively simple to do because of the large numbers of injured children we treated. Most of the principles are applicable both to children and adults, but such details as the size of breathing tubes and the amount of blood to give vary with the condition and size of the child. In a crisis one needs to know these things, as there isn't time to look them up. Judging by the number of reprints requested, these guidelines were very popular in other hospitals and filled a void in many teaching programs.

With the help of Billie Lent, our aggressive and enthusiastic head nurse, I drew up a list of equipment and supplies required in emergency rooms that treat severely injured children. We used it primarily as a checklist when restocking the trauma room after we had turned it into a shambles in the process of resuscitating critically injured children. The list was not an original idea. I had seen a similar one for adults at Parkland Hospital in Dallas in the room where President Kennedy died from bullet wounds. On a whim I sent our list to the editor of the *Journal of Trauma,* a monthly publication read by some fourteen thousand surgeons concerned with caring for the injured. I fully expected a polite rejection and was pleasantly surprised to find our list featured as the lead article a month or two later. It was a simple contribution, but the fact that this widely respected editor had chosen to display it prominently was a hopeful sign. Trauma was at last becoming recognized as the number one threat to the lives and health of children.

43

Trauma

The word trauma means injury. One can suffer either physical or emotional injury, but by itself the word trauma does not have an emotional connotation. It simply means injury. Not long ago, trauma was known as the neglected disease of modern society. Preoccupied as we were with congenital malformations and cancer, and busy looking after hundreds of children with pyloric stenosis, appendicitis, and the like, pediatric surgeons were as guilty as anyone else of neglecting trauma. This is not to say that we did not take good care of the injured children who were brought to us. We did, but the task of conquering this formidable killer demands more of surgeons than the skillful performance of delicate operations.

The first phase of treatment, often as critical to survival as anything that happens later, takes place at the scene of the accident. Trained emergency personnel are seldom the first people to offer assistance. Usually the first to respond are ordinary bystanders who have had no first-aid training. The same is usually true when adults suffer heart attacks. A growing number of lay people have learned cardiopulmonary resuscitation and are able to maintain breathing and circulation for heart attack victims until trained help can be summoned. First-aid measures for the injured are no more complicated. Even young children can learn them, but they must be taught. When professional personnel arrive to take over they must have proper training and the authority to use it. Though not present at the accident scene, the surgeon who initiates and participates in this vital training can greatly influence what happens there.

Critically injured patients require definitive treatment, as distinct from first-aid measures, within the "golden hour," the first sixty minutes after the accident. The mortality goes up by a factor of four when this brief time is exceeded. This means that after a very short period of stabilization they must be quickly transported directly to a trauma center, bypassing community hospitals along the way which are not equipped and staffed to care for them.

The concept of centralized care for critically ill patients is not new, but its application to injured patients has only just begun. Among the first pediatric surgeons to see the need was J. Alex Haller, Chief of Pediatric Surgery at the Johns Hopkins Hospital in Baltimore. There he established the nation's first pediatric trauma center. Using helicopters, the Maryland state police can transport critically injured children directly to the children's trauma center from an accident occurring anywhere in the state. To achieve this goal, Alex spent countless hours conferring with state and local government officials and integrating his pediatric trauma center into the comprehensive Maryland Emergency Medical System. He and Dr. R. Adams Cowley, who directs the system, were greatly aided in their early efforts by Governor Marvin Mandel, himself an accident victim who owes his life to prompt, well-organized trauma care. Without close cooperation between surgeons and government officials effective trauma-care systems do not develop. The surgeon, who sees the need, must initiate the dialogue and work long and hard to sustain it.

Beyond establishing trauma centers and the rescue and transport systems that support them there is much more to be done. Medical students and physicians at all levels, as well as nurses and paramedical personnel, require more training in the care of the injured than ever was provided before. Surgeons are beginning to devote more time to professional education, and most of them find the effort very rewarding.

During the past twenty years research has produced spectacular improvement in the care of burned children, but advances in treating other kinds of injuries have been hampered by lack of funding. There has been very little support for research in human behavior, wherein lie many valuable clues to accident prevention. For every federal dollar spent on research in cancer and heart disease, less than a penny has been spent on trauma research.

Concerned as they may be with the many problems of injury, surgeons cannot hope to make impressive inroads if they work in a vacuum. Not only must they relate to their medical colleagues and their allies in nursing and related professions, but they must deal effectively with police, fire, and ambulance personnel, health departments and government officials. Most important, they must involve the public.

The success of the American Heart Association and the American Cancer Society dramatically illustrate what can be done when physicians pool their efforts with those of an informed public. Physicians found that if they took time to explain and interpret their medical knowledge to lay people, these laymen and women could achieve objectives that the medical profession could not. Physicians working alone could not hope to accomplish the monumental tasks of public education and fund raising which were essential to success. There are only three hundred eleven thousand physicians in active practice in the United States. The American Heart Association and the American Cancer Society each claim over two million volunteers. Every year these two vast armies of volunteers raise over a hundred million dollars for research, public and professional education, and community service. In doing so they have educated the public. The average citizen has been alerted to the dangers of heart disease and cancer, whereas he still does not fully realize the importance of injury as the major threat to his children and does not see a clear role for himself in helping to bring it under control.

It required more than fifty years for the lessons of these two huge voluntary health agencies to be translated into the founding of a similar organization to deal with trauma. Like the others, the American Trauma Society was founded by a small group of concerned physicians. In this case they were surgeons, led by Dr. Jonathan Rhoads, who had served as president of the American Cancer Society. Gradually more and more lay people began to participate. Initial funding came from a few small grants and from physicians and lay people who were willing to become founding members. At a national meeting of pediatric surgeons I called upon my colleagues to join and support the fledgling organization. Their response was nearly unanimous, and on the basis of their support I was placed on the national board of directors and soon thereafter on the executive committee of the Trauma Society.

Like the two organizations after which ours was patterned, we attempted to establish divisions in every state and units in major cities, rural districts, and individual communities. Had we realized the magnitude of the task we might never have begun it. Physicians tended to understand what we were trying to do, and enlisting their aid was relatively easy. It was much more difficult to convince lay people, particularly busy, influential community leaders, that their efforts really could make a difference. Two who did see opportunities to contribute were Archie Boe and Richard Ogilvie. Mr. Boe was chairman of Allstate Insurance, the largest provider of automobile insurance in the country. Mr. Ogilvie, the ex-governor of Illinois, was, like Governor Mandel, the victim of a serious injury and owes his life to timely, skilled trauma care. Shortly after joining us, he became our chairman.

Quite naturally, we wanted to do everything at once. We wanted divisions and units everywhere. We wanted trauma centers. We wanted better ambulances with better equipment and better trained people to man them. We wanted a nationwide program of professional education. We wanted to be able to raise money for badly needed research. We wanted an organization that could work effectively with government officials at all levels. We wanted the public to understand and help us. More than one skeptical businessman told us our goals were too broad to accomplish all at once.

When we finally ordered our priorities and narrowed our immediate goals to fostering trauma centers, we began to make more headway. Today we are focusing our efforts upon alerting the public to the importance of centralized care for the critically injured and upon convincing them that if enough people want better trauma care in their communities they can have it.

In a few communities, notably in Maryland, Washington, D.C., Wisconsin, Illinois, Pennsylvania, and California, the

American Trauma Society has become recognized and loyally supported. When we compare our meager accomplishments to those of the Heart Association and the Cancer Society our progress seems painfully slow. Members of these organizations are quick to point out that they enjoy a fifty-year head start and that their early progress was not rapid either. The Trauma Society is in its infancy, but the need for it is valid and its growth and success are inevitable. Having served as its president from 1975 to 1978, I have seen firsthand what it can accomplish. The average citizen has inherent desires to help himself, protect his family, and help others. To satisfy these needs, enormous numbers of people respond to education with a generous outpouring of time, talents, and money to support education, research, and an organized system for care of the injured. In areas where this system is well developed, the saving of life and reduction of disability are truly remarkable. An admiring nation followed the progress of President Reagan and his press secretary, James Brady, who were transported at once to the trauma center at George Washington University where they received expert definitive treatment within minutes of injury. Surely injured children everywhere deserve no less.

44

A Gift of Courage

By now we had been in Columbus nearly twenty years and it was time to go home to New England. My life in Columbus had been a series of wonderful experiences. What made them wonderful was the close relationships that came to me as a children's surgeon—relationships with doctors and nurses, with hundreds of brave and anxious mothers and fathers, and most of all, with children. What experience had been most rewarding? Which child had most successfully wormed his way into my heart? I think it was Tommy Burr.

I've wondered many, many times why Tommy's story ended the way it did. I think it would have ended differently had I not been witness to the lighting of a little candle many years ago.

When I was twelve years old, I went away to boarding school in a small town in New England. My most vivid memory of that first year away from home was of the candlelight vesper service on the last Sunday evening before Christmas. The school was on the side of a hill overlooking the Deerfield Valley. At five o'clock in the afternoon all the boys and all the masters gathered together and walked down through the gathering darkness to a little church in the village below. Waiting for us there was the minister, whom I remember as the oldest man I'd ever seen and very, very wise. As we entered the church, everything was dark except for one candle which the old gentleman held in his hand. One by one we boys lighted our candles from his, and soon the whole church was warm and bright with candlelight. When we were all in our places, he held up the one little candle from which all that light had come and said, "Boys, as one light lights another nor grows less, so nobleness enkindles nobleness." And then we sang some Christmas carols and blew out our candles and walked back up the hill to school. As I tramped up the hill through the snow that winter's night when I was twelve years old, I thought "nobleness enkindling nobleness" was the greatest idea in all the world.

I first met Tommy Burr in the spring of 1966, when he was ten years old. He had been admitted to the Children's Hospital because his blood pressure was much too high. After a series of exhaustive tests, we found that Tommy's problem was caused by a pheochromocytoma, a rare tumor of the adrenal gland which produces huge quantities of adrenalin. Most pheochromocytomas are not malignant, but all of them must be removed before the overproduction of adrenalin drives the blood pressure up to levels incompatible with life. Removing a pheochromocytoma is not ordinarily a very difficult task, but this was no ordinary patient, for in addition to his pheochromocytoma Tommy Burr had hemophilia.

The clotting of blood is a complex process that is dependent upon the interaction of a number of different substances. The substance of which hemophiliacs are deficient is known as Factor VIII. All hemophiliacs are capable of making their own Factor VIII, but they do so at a pitifully slow rate. In the blood of those most severely affected, Factor VIII seldom rises above 5 percent of the normal level. The ultimate conquest of hemophilia will come from an answer to the questions, "Why, if they can make Factor VIII, do they do so so slowly?" and "What can be done to accelerate this abnormally slow production?" But all that lies in the future. So far, no one has been able to influence the rate of Factor VIII production, and no one has been able to make the substance synthetically. The treatment of all hemophiliacs still rests, as it always has, upon supplying them in their hours of crisis with Factor VIII from the blood of normal people.

The simplest method is the transfusion of fresh whole blood. Using fresh whole blood, minor injuries can be brought under control, and the simplest of operations can be performed. Factor VIII deteriorates rapidly when blood is stored in a blood bank, and once transfused to a patient, half of the factor is gone within four hours. For all but very minor wounds, transfusion of fresh whole blood must be repeated every four hours for about two weeks as the wound goes through the early phases of healing. The limiting factor soon becomes the availability of compatible donors who are willing to have their blood drawn at such odd hours as midnight or four o'clock in the morning.

The first great advance came from the recognition that the factor resides in the plasma, or liquid portion of the blood. The red blood cells can be discarded or used for other purposes. With the red cells removed, plasma can be frozen, and in the frozen state the factor retains its potency for many months. This allows the advance collection and stockpiling of Factor VIII against emergencies and greatly simplifies the management of the donors.

Using fresh-frozen plasma, such operations as appendectomy can be performed with relative safety and some much more complicated procedures have been performed. As far as we know, no one has ever removed a pheochromocytoma from a hemophiliac boy using either fresh whole blood, fresh-frozen plasma, or a combination of the two. As the complexity of the operation increases, the need for Factor VIII increases, and the limiting factor becomes the volume of plasma required to contain it. If too much plasma is given too rapidly, the patient literally drowns in his own and other people's juices.

Since no one was able to influence the rate of Factor VIII production and no one was able to produce it synthetically, all research efforts in the 1960s were devoted toward finding ways to concentrate the factor so that it could be given in a smaller volume of plasma. Two years before Tommy's tumor was discovered, a remarkable accident took place in California which was to change forever the outlook for boys with this dread disease. While giving a hemophiliac patient a transfusion of fresh-frozen plasma from a transparent plastic bag, Dr. Judith Pool happened to notice that there was a small amount of white precipitate in the bottom of the bag. This sort of precipitate was never seen when fresh-frozen plasma was thawed quickly. Dr.

Pool reasoned correctly that the precipitate was the result of rapid freezing followed by accidentally slow thawing, and she set about trying to discover what it was made of. To her intense delight, she found that it was very rich in Factor VIII. During the next two years she perfected and published her method of cryoprecipitation, or precipitation with the use of cold, by which the Factor VIII from a pint of blood can be concentrated into less than an ounce of plasma.

Armed with this new information, we set about planning an attack on Tommy's tumor. The equipment necessary for the cryoprecipitation process was in very short supply. The Red Cross blood bank on Broad Street was able to acquire only enough of it to process four pints of blood at a time. This imposed serious limitations on the donors, for large groups of them could not simply wander down to the blood bank on their lunch hour to give a pint of blood. The bloodmobile, which accommodates the donors by going to their place of employment, could not be used because of the delays involved. Every pint had to be donated at the main blood bank on Broad Street according to a strict schedule so that it could be started immediately through the cryoprecipitation process before any of the precious Factor VIII began to deteriorate. The Red Cross assigned two technicians full time to this project, and in about three weeks they had assembled and processed two hundred pints of blood.

The cryoprecipitation process was not refined enough to allow the use of different blood types. Every donor had to have the same blood type as the patient. Tommy's blood type was B positive, a type shared by only 12 percent of the normal population. When you eliminate everyone who is too old to give, everyone who is too young, everyone who has given too recently to be allowed to give again, and everyone with a history of hepatitis, anemia, or other disqualifying conditions, you can see that in order to obtain two hundred pints of acceptable B-positive blood, the Red Cross must have communicated effectively with more than two thousand people who, were they acceptable in every way, would have been willing to come down by appointment to the main blood bank on Broad Street to give a pint of blood for a little boy they had never seen.

This was a communications task of no small magnitude. It

could never have been accomplished without the effort of someone like Carolyn Focht, a young reporter for the Columbus *Dispatch*. She came to Children's Hospital, talked with Tommy and his parents, and wrote the first of a series of forty-five consecutive articles and news items which were to win for her a coveted national award for the best medical journalism of 1966. The magnitude of Carolyn's contribution, and that of the radio and television personalities who joined her later, could be appreciated only in retrospect. When the final count was made, the two hundred pints of blood we thought would see Tommy through his operation and through every conceivable complication turned out to be a drop in the bucket. Before we desisted from our efforts to save his life, we had used five times two hundred pints of blood!

The day of the operation finally came. While the anesthetists were putting Tommy to sleep, I saw with my own eyes for the first time the significance of Dr. Pool's discovery, as we gave him in four ounces of plasma the concentrated Factor VIII from a whole gallon of blood. Through a long transverse incision we entered his abdomen and there at the upper pole of the right kidney, just where the x-rays had shown it would be, was a rounded purplish tumor about the size of a plum. We divided the blood vessels and lifted it away with no more difficulty than one would have had with the average gallbladder. Before his incision was closed his blood pressure, which had been abnormally high for weeks, had started to fall toward the normal range. As we wheeled him into the recovery room we commented to each other on what a remarkable substance this concentrated Factor VIII must be, for we had had no more difficulty with bleeding than if we had operated upon a perfectly normal boy.

Now the long vigil began. During every hour of every day and night for two long weeks we must keep his Factor VIII above a critical level. If we allowed it to drop too low, even momentarily, a sudden motion or a fit of coughing might precipitate a hemorrhage that could be impossible to stop. The rate at which we administered Factor VIII was governed by a special clotting test, which was performed by two technicians, Ruth Johnson and Linda Fear. These two women took Tommy on as a special project, and abandoning all ideas of an eight-hour shift, divided up the week in such a fashion that one or the other of them was always in the hospital, usually not far from Tommy's bedside.

Monday, Monday night, Tuesday, Tuesday night—all went well, but on Wednesday at three o'clock in the morning my telephone rang with the dreaded news that Tommy was bleeding. When I arrived at his bedside I found Linda Fear standing beside him with tears streaming down her face. She had checked and double checked every test that had been performed since his operation, and every one of them was normal. Provided no mistakes had been made, this was extremely important information. If his blood was clotting normally a surgeon might hope to reenter his abdomen and find a bleeding vessel which could be ligated. If his clotting was not normal, surgical intervention could only aggravate his problem and might very easily kill him. We decided that Linda and her information had to be trusted, and just as the sun came up we returned to the operating room to try to find the bleeding vessel. Gently and carefully we wiped away the blood —but we found no bleeding vessel. For reasons totally obscure to us the bleeding had stopped all by itself, and we were forced to close his abdomen without having been able to do anything to prevent it from starting up again in the future.

We decided that our best hope lay in beginning a new fourteen-day program administering Factor VIII at twice our previous rate. This would require Factor VIII from twenty-four donors a day. The remains of our original two hundred units, which only two days ago had seemed an inexhaustible supply, now would last less than a week. Again, Carolyn Focht put out the call for donors and again, from every corner of the city, the donors came.

This time things went smoothly for a week, and then at three o'clock in the morning Tommy started bleeding even faster than before. The clotting tests were normal, and we returned to the operating room under emergency conditions to try once more to find the bleeding vessel. Again, we were thwarted. Just as mysteriously as it had started, the bleeding had stopped all by itself. Disappointed and frustrated, we closed his abdomen and called a council of war to try to decide what to do next. We concluded that even though all of his clotting tests had been normal, we must have allowed his Factor VIII level to fall too low. On that basis we decided to start all over again with a new fourteen-day program, doubling the frequency with which we performed our clotting tests and doubling the rate at which we gave him Factor VIII.

Now we would require forty-eight B-positive donors a day. The Red Cross blood bank on Broad Street, for the first and only time except in time of war, was kept open twenty-four hours a day, seven days a week to receive and process the blood from B-positive donors. Chet Long, Hugh DeMoss, and other personalities of radio and television joined Carolyn in spreading the word of our need, and although we saw the bottom of the barrel once or twice, we never quite ran out.

During the days and nights that followed this second futile operation, I was plagued with the question, "What could I, or any surgeon, do if the bleeding started again?" I asked for advice from everyone I could think of, both in my own hospital and in others across the country. The advice I got was remarkably simple, "Don't try a third time an operation that already has failed twice. Perhaps if you just let the bleeding continue, the pressure within his abdomen will build up high enough to stop the bleeding." It didn't seem like very good advice to me, but it came from everyone I asked. With uneasy apprehension I settled down to wait out the critical fourteen days.

Hour after hour, day after day, the anxious watch wore on. The burden of this constant vigil bore heavily down upon the two technicians who were doing all of Tommy's clotting tests. By Monday morning, as our marathon entered its fourth week, Ruth Johnson had become so exhausted that her physician would not let her come to work. Without a murmur Linda Fear, who already had been on duty for twelve hours, moved into the hospital to stay with us around the clock as long as she was needed.

Monday, Monday night, Tuesday, Tuesday night, Wednesday —twelve days had gone by without bleeding. The wound was nearly healed; the long watch was nearly over. Mrs. Burr and I were standing by his bedside when we saw the fateful look upon his face. It was the look which down through the ages has cast terror into the hearts of mothers of boys with hemophilia, a look which says more poignantly than any words can tell, "Help me, help me, Mother, I'm bleeding!"

I never felt so helpless in all my life as I did that night watching his little abdomen fill up with blood. Maybe, I thought, just maybe it will work. Maybe the pressure will build up high enough to tamponade the bleeding vessel—but I really didn't think it would. I did not have long to wonder because suddenly at midnight the bandage overlying his incision turned red with blood, and my heart almost stopped as I realized what this meant! The edges of his incision were coming apart! Now there would be no way to contain the blood, no way for pressure to build up and tamponade the bleeding. Finally at four o'clock in the morning I admitted to myself what others had been trying to tell me for hours. We were defeated. Nothing we had tried had worked. Tommy was dying. There was nothing new to try.

I climbed the stairs with a heavy heart to thank Linda and tell her she could go home. How could I thank her? What could I say to her? She had been with us around the clock since Sunday evening. I opened the door to her little laboratory and there she sat, on the edge of a makeshift cot, in a crumpled uniform she had put on three days and now almost four full nights before. In one hand she held a test tube containing a solution to which she had added a few drops of Tommy's blood. In the other hand she held a stopwatch, counting the seconds until the appearance of the first fine strands of clot. When they did appear, well within the normal time limit, she stopped the stopwatch with a force I thought would surely shatter it and said, "Come on, Tommy, hang on!" With awesome clarity I saw in Linda's weary eyes the flickering of the little candle I had seen so many years ago, and I knew that she was right. He wasn't oozing to death because he had hemophilia. The clotting substance we were giving him was working. His blood was clotting just as normally as any other little boy's. There had to be something wrong beneath his incision, and I had to be able to find it! With no new tricks up my sleeve, against the best advice I'd been given, I took him back to the operating room and for the third time reopened his incision. Gently and carefully, as we had done before, we wiped away the blood and suddenly *there it was!* With every beat of his heart a tiny jet of blood spurted from the mouth of an untied vessel. We clamped and tied the bleeding artery, and he never bled again.

Three weeks later, having used 960 pints of blood, Tommy Burr put on his clothes and went home. As I watched him go I felt a thrill the likes of which I know will never come to me again. I wondered then, for the first of many, many times, "What caused this precious miracle?" Was it science, enabling us to identify the substance missing from his blood? Was it luck, favoring the prepared mind of Dr. Pool, allowing her to snatch the seeds of a great discovery from the wreckage of a careless accident? Was it the skill, devotion, and teamwork of all of the people at Children's Hospital who worked so hard for him? Surely this marathon had brought out the best in many, many people. Was it communication—the newspapers, radio, and television—that had alerted a whole city to his need and brought a thousand people with the right blood type to stand patiently in line to give a pint of blood for a little boy they had never even seen? Was it prayer? Later we learned that prayers were said for Tommy every Sunday in more than sixty churches. Was it something within the little boy himself? Truly, he did have a gallant heart. Or was it a gift of courage glowing for me in Linda's tired eyes that dreary morning when I thought all hope had gone?

Index

Morse at
  emergency medicine, 299–305
  first patients, 163–68
  kidney transplantations, 238–68
  most rewarding case, 311–19
  patient's office, 170–72
  supervising of patients' care,
    204–5
  surgical teaching, 189–94, 237
  threatened with malpractice
    suit, 295–98
Columbus *Dispatch*, 315
Computerized axial tomography
    (CAT), 294
Congenital intestinal obstruction,
    189–94, 200, 205
Congenital malformations, 73–74, 78,
    308
Consciousness, loss of, 303–4
Constipation, 172–74
Coombs' test, 40
Cornea transplantation, 238
Cornell Medical School, 2–7, 8
Cotter, Walter, 79–85
Crafoord, Dr., 88, 93
Crandon, John, 56, 126, 143
Cremaster, 103, 104
Crompton, Helen, 170–76, 295–96
Cryoprecipitation, 314
Curley, James Michael, 125, 142–43,
    161
Cyanosis, 90

Debricin, 136, 137, 228
Defensive medicine, 294, 298
Deterling, Ralph, 143–45, 155–56,
    158, 159
Diabetes, 24–26, 267
Diabetic coma, 118
Dialysis, 238, 239, 241, 244, 246, 250,
    252, 257, 258, 268
Dialyzers, 239–42, 245, 246, 256
Diarrhea
  fulminating, 26
  infant, 73
Diamond, Dr., 32–34, 36, 38
Diaphragmatic hernias, 73
Digitalis, 47, 48
Doan, Dean Charles, 149, 155
Down's syndrome, 289–92
Drugs
  anticancer, 168, 282, 283

  See also names of drugs
Ductus arteriosus, 86–87
Dunphy, J. Englebert, 49, 62
Duodenal atresia, 289, 290, 292
Duodenum, 273, 274, 277

Economopoulis, Chris, 67–68, 127,
    141
Electrocardiograms, 21–22, 47, 48
Electroencephalograms, 255
Emergency medicine, 299–305
Empyema, 163–64
Encephalograms, 252
Enemas, 173–74
Epiphyseal injuries, 121–22
Erythroblastosis, 37–39, 41, 272
Erythroblasts, 37
Erythromycin, 163
Esophageal atresia, 177–80, 198
Esophageal replacement, 109, 113
Esophageal varices, 113, 274
Esophagus, 177, 178, 198
  abnormalities of, 107–14
Ethical decisions, 288–92

Factor VIII, 312–17
Fallopian tubes, 215
Fallot, tetralogy of, 90
Farber, Sidney, 28–32, 73, 166, 168,
    280
Fear, Linda, 315–19
Fernald, Will, 176–80
Flammable sleepwear, 230
Floating Hospital, 126, 144, 146
Flynn, J. Edward, 55, 126
Focht, Carolyn, 315, 316, 317
Fractures, 120–24
Frank, Chuck, 269–70
Frye, Tom, 218–19, 237, 260, 277,
    304
Funnel chest. *See* Pectus excavatum

Gallbladder, 273, 277, 315
Gastroenteritis, 212
Gastrostomy tube, 108, 178, 179, 180
Gellis, Sidney, 19, 69, 125–26, 146
George Washington University
    trauma center, 310
German measles, 190
Graham, Dr., 244, 250, 251, 253, 256
Greenough, Janice, 48
Gridiron incision, 209

Nephrologists, 255–56
Neuroblastoma, 282
Neurosurgery, 71–72, 78–85, 217, 294–95
New England Journal of Medicine, 124
New England Surgical Society, 153
Newton, Bill, 168, 281, 283
Night float, 45–46
Non-flammable sleepwear, 230
North Shore Babies' Hospital, 45
Novocain, 301
Nursemaid's elbow, 122
Nutrition, 216
  burned patients and, 230

Ohio State University, 149, 161, 162, 267
Omentum, 213
Oncologists, 281, 283
Open heart surgery, 117
Orthopedists, 217
Osler, Sir William, 10
Osteomyelitis, 123
Oxygenators, 91–92

Patent ductus arteriosus, 21, 86–93
Pathology, 65
Pearson, Art, 244, 245, 250–53, 255–56, 259–62, 267
Pectus excavatum, 128–31, 198
Pediatric cardiology, 46–47
Pediatric training programs, 51–52
Pediatric trauma center, 307, 309
Penicillin, 10, 73, 123–24, 163, 213, 225
Pentothal, 208
Peritoneum, 102, 187, 209
Peritonitis, 200, 212–15
Pernicious anemia, 44
Peter Bent Brigham Hospital, 72, 244
Pheochromocytoma, 312–19
Pineal glioma, 83
Platelets, 28, 32
Pneumonia, 73, 177
Poliomyelitis, 79–80
Pontocaine, 63, 64, 65
Pool, Judith, 313–15, 319
Portal hypertension, 113
Potts, Willis, 90, 91
Pratt, Edwin, 15–16

Prednisone, 248, 251, 254, 265, 267
  side effects of, 264–65
Premature babies, 12–13, 24–25
Processus vaginalis, 102
Pulmonary artery, 86, 87, 90
Pulmonary edema, 226
Pulmonic stenosis, 90
Pyloric canal, 188
Pyloric stenosis, 183–88, 204, 306
Pylorus, 183–84, 187

Radiation, 286, 287
Radioactive isotope scan, 297–98
Radiologists, 193, 295
Radiotherapists, 281, 282, 283
Ravitch, Mark, 200–1, 233
Red blood cells, 28, 37–38, 313
Red Cross blood bank, 314, 317
Respirators, 216, 288
Retrolental fibroplasia, 13
Rh babies, 35–42
Rheumatic fever, 9–10, 12, 46
Rh factor, 36–42
Rh incompatibility, 272
Rh negative red blood cells, 38–42
Rh positive red blood cells, 38–42
Rickets, 19
Rowe, Marc, 219, 237
Royal Children's Hospital (Melbourne), 198
Ruptured spleen, 218
Rupture of the appendix, 212–15

St. Vitus' dance. *See* Rheumatic fever
Salk, Jonas, 79
Santulli, Tom, 189
Sayers, Martin Peter, 217, 246, 304
Scribner shunts, 257–59
Scrotum, 102, 103
Scrub nurses, 54, 56
Seconal, 106, 174, 207, 212
Sellors, Holmes, 90, 91
Seymour, Miner, 299–300
Shock, 225
Silastic tubing, 257, 258
Skin grafts, 133, 227–28, 230
Smith, John P. (JP), 217–23, 224, 237, 240, 243, 247, 252, 256, 260–62, 266, 267
Sodium pentothal, 208
Spermatic cord, 102, 103, 105